·H·E·A·L·I·N·G·
ENVIRONMENTS

·H·E·A·L·I·N·G·

ENVIRONMENTS

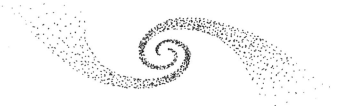

Your Guide to Indoor Well-Being

CAROL VENOLIA

Foreword by Debra Lynn Dadd

Illustrations by Roberta DeVaul

CELESTIAL ARTS
Berkeley, California

CELESTIAL ARTS
P.O. Box 7327
Berkeley, California 94707

Cover design by Ken Scott
Text design by Nancy Austin
Composition by The Recorder Typesetting Network
Illustrations © 1988 by Roberta DeVaul

Library of Congress Cataloging in Publication Data

Venolia, Carol, 1951-
Healing environments: your guide to indoor well-being / Carol Venolia:
foreword by Debra Lynn Dadd.
p. cm.
Bibliography: p.
Includes index.
ISBN 0-89087-497-2
1. Architecture—Health aspects. 2. Architecture—Psychological
aspects. I. Title.
RA566.6.V46 1988
720—dc19

ISBN 0-89087-497-2

First Printing, 1988

Manufactured in the United States of America

3   4   5   —   96   95   94   93

· TABLE · OF · CONTENTS ·

· III · SYNTHESIS ·

· ACKNOWLEDGMENTS ·

Now I know why authors lavish so much gratitude on their friends and colleagues at the beginning of each book. It's true; the community of support that made this book what it is deserves deep appreciation and recognition.

First, I thank and salute my publisher, Dave Hinds of Celestial Arts, for picking up the spark of this book and breathing life into it; his faith in the project was pivotal to its growth. Warm thanks, too, to Paul Reed of Celestial for caringly editing and turning the manuscript into a book, to Nancy Austin who deftly expressed the spirit of this book through its design, and to Ken Scott for his superb cover art.

In the course of writing *Healing Environments*, several people provided valuable information and feedback. Much of Chapter 2, Health and Place, is the product of discussions with Keith Kroeber. Zee and Ed Randegger of *Environ* magazine were tireless in providing me information, suggestions, and encouragement. Constance McKnight, who could have written this book herself, was generous with resources, appropriate criticism, and moral support. Architect Denise Owen contributed needed insights between early versions of the manuscript.

Debra Lynn Dadd kindly agreed to introduce this book to you via her Foreword and gave valuable feedback on the text. John Reynolds, Professor of Environmental Control Systems at the University of Oregon Department of Architecture, found time in a busy schedule to make suggestions for the chapters on light, sound, and the thermal environment; John also deserves appreciation for encouraging me to follow my own instincts as his architecture student—instincts that eventually lead to *Healing Environments*.

Stuart Chudnofsky, M.D., made comments on Chapter 11, Indoor Air Quality, that contributed to its revision. Gail Brager, Associate Professor of Architecture at the University of California at

Berkeley, also provided me with volumes of valuable information on Indoor Air Quality. And Bobbi DeVaul Thiede poured her heart into the illustrations.

A special tribute is due to Cristina Ismael. Her book, *The Healing Environment,* stood alone in its field for over a decade and was a major source of inspiration for this book.

Many others inspired, taught, informed, and lovingly corrected me in creating *Healing Environments.* Engineer Barbara Atkinson, healer Leah Garfield, therapist Betty Eilerman, Richard Feather Anderson of the Westcoast Institute of Sacred Ecology, Mike Luttrell of Warm Floors, Fred and Cheryl Mitouer of the Pacific School of Massage, architect Steve Sheldon, builder Charles Morgan, Joan Westcott, Helen Garcia, Debra Carroll, Kersten Tanner, Judith Fisher, Gina Ryerson, Anita Hill, Marjorie and Jim Mills, Jasmin Clower, Mark Mendell, Susan Molloy, and Derek Hoyle are all a part of this book.

Most of all, I thank my parents, Jan and Wayne Venolia, for multitudinous large and small acts of support. They provided substantive input, editorial suggestions, moral support, computer consultation, and clerical help.

Everyone named here has my heartfelt gratitude, but none are to be blamed for my decisions about what to include and what to leave out.

Finally, I am grateful for all my friends and neighbors in Gualala, Point Arena, and The Sea Ranch, who constantly inquired about the state of my book, suggested new resources, tolerated my "writer's mood swings," and encouraged me at every turn. My love and thanks to you all; the best healing environment is a community of friends!

· FOREWORD ·

by Debra Lynn Dadd

For years I limited my definition of "healing environment" to "an environment that doesn't make me physically ill—that doesn't contain substances or materials known to be toxic or harmful." With this view I wrote two books on natural alternatives to household toxics*, published a newsletter, wrote magazine articles, gave lectures, made media appearances, and bought a house which I diligently renovated until it was the epitome of nontoxic living.

But something was missing. While I filled my house with objects I liked, it wasn't really a *home*. While almost everything I had was made from natural materials, there was no connection with the cycles and spirit of nature. Although my self-made habitat healed my body, it did nothing to nourish my soul.

I began to research other aspects of the indoor environment— light, sound, color, temperature, energy—and finally realized that the one factor my house lacked most was any sort of connection to its immediate surroundings. It was placed in the land and built as if the earth around it were an asphalt parking lot instead of the thriving forest it was. As I became more and more aware of all the different factors involved in creating an integrated environment that would nurture body, mind, and spirit, I realized that my present house could not be adequately altered to meet my needs. I sold it with the idea that I would take some time living in different places, then buy some land and build.

I had always had a desire to visit England, and this seemed to be a good time to go. I wanted to experience living in a different culture, to get new ideas and to gain more clarity on what was important to me at home. When Carol told me about this book, it sounded like the guide I needed to help me re-evaluate what I wanted in the place that I live. So two days before I was to get on the plane

---

Nontoxic and Natural and *The Nontoxic Home* (see Bibliography).

to London, I asked Carol to send her manuscript to me. As I read it in my hotel room, one rainy day in Cornwall, I saw that Carol had in fact compiled, in a complete and usable form, all the factors I needed to consider to create my perfect home. *Healing Environments* touches on subjects I had not included in my previous view— but now saw as necessary parts to create a whole indoor environment. Her Awareness Exercises throughout the book triggered interesting observations for me about my own sense of home.

As I traveled throughout the British Isles, I had plenty of opportunity to experience different environments, to see what I felt "comfortable" with. I also wanted to know if there was anything I missed about my previous house that I wanted to include in my new home. The answer to that question came quickly: my cotton flannel sheets and pillowcases, feather pillows, down comforter, featherbeds, fuzzy wool mattress pad . . . if I could only have my natural bedding, it almost wouldn't matter where I slept.

The concept of "healing environment" stayed with me, and on my trip I kept my awareness open for places that felt healing to me. I found one while standing in the center of an ancient sacred stone circle, feeling the concentrated enlightening energy of the place that had drawn people to the spot for centuries. Another appeared as I transformed a dreary hotel room one evening, by simply lighting a candle. One day I climbed to the top of a mountain on an island in the Outer Hebrides, and as the north wind blew straight through my down parka, I was healed by the thought of going back to California (where it was warm, at least!) and finding my new home.

Now, as I write this, I'm sitting in a tiny room with not much more than bed, desk, and bookshelves. I'm living in the city with the rooftop of the next building out my window and four housemates who seem always to be taking showers at the same time I want to. But, still, this is a very healing environment for me, because I'm active, in motion, progressing, thinking, and loving.

Part of my becoming a more loving person is to interact more lovingly with my environment. After spending years focusing only on what goes on within the four walls that surround me, I now see that what goes on within those four walls always has an effect on what happens beyond them. *Healing Environments* brings this connection home and shows how we can create buildings that nurture ourselves, and the Earth as well.

·H·E·A·L·I·N·G·
ENVIRONMENTS

· I ·

B·A·C·K·G·R·O·U·N·D·

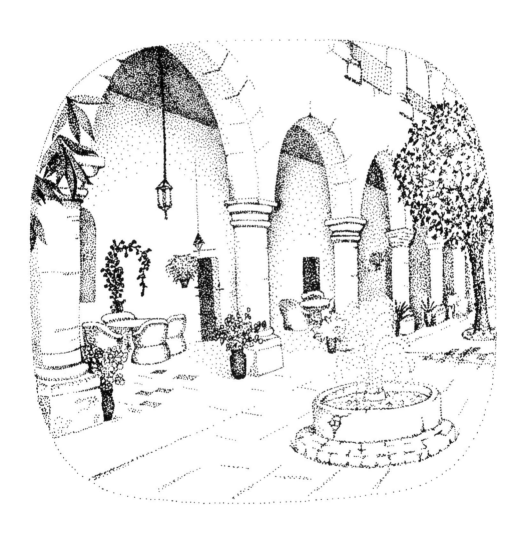

· CHAPTER · 1 ·

Welcome

If you live indoors and care about your health, this book is for you. It will take you on a journey of self-exploration and increase your knowledge about your intimate relationships with buildings. Whatever your current state of health, you will learn how the buildings you inhabit can influence your mental, physical, and emotional well-being. And you will learn how to bring your indoor environment—new or old, rented or owned—into greater harmony with life, steadily improving your health.

Many of us consciously pursue good health, but we often overlook the powerful role of our immediate physical environment. Each of us has a close, evolving relationship with the places where we live, work, and otherwise spend our time. We interact with our surroundings through all of our senses. We make changes in our environment, and it in turn influences our lives. Places limit us, challenge us, expand us, support us, bore us, and excite us. Every aspect of these interactions becomes a part of our total well-being, often in subtle, unexamined ways.

There are as many ways of looking at health and place as there are of looking at health itself. Just as you, an individual, encompass a wide range of aspects, you and your environment relate to each other on multiple levels. Your surroundings not only have physical components that influence your health (such as toxicity of materials, relative humidity, or light quality), they also have "mental" qualities (the message content of an imposing government building, for example), and "emotional" aspects (the way a place feels)—all of which contribute to your total state. You, in turn, are constantly responding to the place you're in, physically, mentally, emotionally, and spiritually.

Buildings are nearly always in the background, so we tend to be unaware of how powerfully they interact with us—rather like subliminal messages. And when buildings frustrate, limit, or even poison us, we may take these effects for granted; we forget how good we could feel without such burdens. As long as buildings are a dominant factor in our lives, and as long as new ones are going up every day, we might as well learn how to do them right.

You are neither the victim nor the master of your environment. You are partners with it in a multi-dimensional dance. You push, you yield; you are yielded to, you are pushed on. And, ultimately, you come to know that you and your environment are one.

This book could legitimately touch on every aspect of life, and each subject could fill a book in itself. To avoid tedium, the measuring rod for what's included in this book is *you.* You will learn about things you can do and attitudes you can develop that will effect health-supporting changes in your surroundings—actions you can take without rallying masses in support, waiting for a government agency to hear you, or changing the course of industry. My aim is to cover each subject well enough to increase your awareness of its role in your health, to give you basic tools for dealing with it, and to point you in the direction of more information. But most of all, I want to tie the subjects together into an encompassing frame of reference.

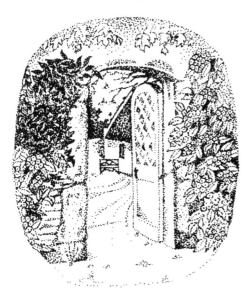

When we bring our environments into greater harmony with life, we set healing forces in motion that carry into every part of our lives. The title *Healing Environments* is a conscious *double entendre.* Not only is it important that we find or make places that are healing to us, but it matters that we be healers of places as well. As we strengthen ourselves in our healing homes and workplaces, and as we discover our own capabilities as creators of positive change, we begin to widen our sphere of influence. Each time we heal an aspect of our environment, we not only increase our vitality, but we also bring that healing to others. As we heighten our awareness of healing environments, we will more readily perceive places outside our immediate sphere that feel alive as well as places that need healing. Though this book focuses on individuals and small groups, there is no real boundary between the "person scale" and the "planet scale." There is no such thing as health for the individual without health for the region and the whole earth. Conversely, I believe that the planet cannot be healed by people who are not healing themselves. It starts with us. The self-determination you gain by increasing your awareness of your surroundings and enlivening them can eventually play out into global healing.

This book is a beginning, an initial offering. I have written it not as an expert, but as an architect with an interest in wholeness, sharing my thoughts and my research so that we may explore and develop our awareness together. Section I introduces basic tools and viewpoints for undertaking this exploration; Section II divides the indoor environment into components so that we can consider them in more depth; and Section III ties the components together into healing attitudes and applications.

Don't just read this book. Get involved with it; keep a notebook of the insights you have as you move through it. Be playful—include sketches, photos, found objects. You'll be surprised and gratified as a new picture of yourself in the world emerges. To help with this process, you will find Awareness Exercises in most chapters set off in italics. They are your key to making the most powerful use of this book by plumbing your depths for inspiration and tailoring the material to you. The more you let yourself get into these exercises, the more you will get out of the book—and the more vital will be your environmental healing.

When you come to an Awareness Exercise, I suggest that you stop reading for a moment, slow down, make sure you're physically comfortable, let your breathing become deep and relaxed, and then turn your attention to the exercise. You might find it more effective to have someone read the exercise to you or to tape record it for yourself so that you can concentrate fully; just be sure to leave ample pauses between the suggestions or questions. When you finish the exercise, record your experiences in your notebook; they'll become increasingly useful as you proceed.

If you don't have the time or inclination to do the Awareness Exercises in depth, don't worry; just reading them will expand your perceptions.

I hope that you and the people who share your environments—friends, family, co-workers—will find this book a useful tool for exploration and transformation. Though *Healing Environments* presents a wide range of information and suggestions, it is meant to offer choices, not to overwhelm. Take small steps; the positive feelings they bring you will give you the momentum to carry on to greater steps.

· CHAPTER · 2 ·

Health and Place

*Health is connection and competence in terms
of the whole, which has as its outer limits the earth,
and as its inner limits, the heart.*
—LEONARD DUHL, M.D.

When you are in a healing environment, you know it; no analysis is required. You somehow feel welcome, balanced, and at one with yourself and the world. You are both relaxed and stimulated, reassured and invited to expand. You feel at home.

But though we know healing places when we find them, we're less sure of how to go about making them for ourselves. Places that heal involve an interplay of factors, yet the effect is coherent. We experience the essence of the place, not its parts. But what is that essence? What components go into creating its effect? How can we begin to heal our own environments to help heal ourselves? And what do we mean by "health" and "healing"?

Good health means having the flexibility and the inner resources to respond to both assaults and opportunities. It is more than the absence of disease. We will always be exposed to germs, emotional shocks, and potential physical injuries, but when we are healthy our body and mind rise to meet the challenges. Good health means that we participate in the dynamic web of life; we derive nourishment from the sun, air, water, earth, plants, animals, and people, and we in turn contribute our creativity, labor, vision, and love to them. Health is not a static state of perfection, but a process of interacting with everything around and inside us in ways that promote growth and vitality. In that context, "heal-

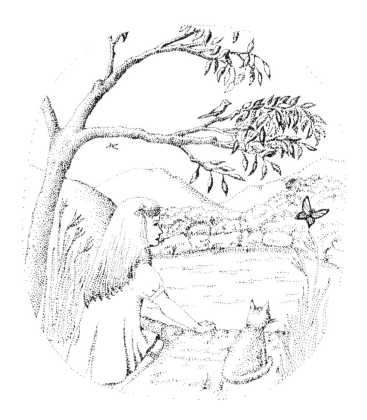

ing" means starting wherever we are now and making incremental changes in our attitudes and actions to encourage health.

What creates this process of health? Medical and psychological researchers agree that self-esteem and a positive outlook are potent factors in our body's ability to resist disease. Though stressors such as family conflict, job dissatisfaction, loss of a loved one, personal failure, overwork, and major life changes lessen our immune responsiveness, our mental reactions to these stressors determine our susceptibility to disease. In other words, people who test high in "psychological vulnerability" (i.e., low in ego strength) become ill after psychological stress more frequently than the average.[1] When we feel low in confidence, helpless to influence the

[1]John B. Jemmott III and Steven E. Locke, M.D., "Psychosocial Factors, Immunologic Mediation, and Human Susceptibility to Infectious Diseases: How Much Do We Know?" *Psychological Bulletin*, Vol. 95, No. 1 (1984), p. 85.

course of our lives, lacking means of self-expression, without a positive vision of our future, and isolated from love and support, we are most likely to succumb to illness. On the other hand, high self-esteem, coping skills, self-expressiveness, an ability to find satisfaction and support, self-awareness, and a feeling that there is a place for us in the world can all increase our resistance to disease. Terminally ill patients who significantly outlive their expectancy tend to be "more creative, more receptive to new ideas, flexible, and argumentative."[2] They are motivated not by a fear of death, but by a desire to be alive and to achieve personally meaningful goals.[3] Medical writer Neville Hodgkinson proposes that "happiness itself is essential to health, and a lack of it is probably the biggest cause of illness and premature death in our society."[4]

A sense of belonging can also make the difference between health and disease. Communities characterized by strong family ties and cultural heritage show lower disease rates and longer life spans than areas marked by rapid change and strong individualism.[5] Numerous studies have found that people with emotional support from family and friends recover from illness more quickly than those who feel isolated or unable to communicate with their families.

Maintaining health requires self-awareness and balance. For example, when we are expending effort our bodies mobilize the "doing" hormones that break down fats and sugars for immediate use.[6] These hormones suppress the hormones that promote growth, renewal, repair, and the maintenance of the body's defenses. When we are aware of our inner cues, we naturally alternate periods of activity and stress with periods of self-nurturing so that our bodies have a chance to replenish themselves. Balance is needed, too, between self-assertiveness and cooperation, determination and flexibility, and the expression of authority and the willingness to adapt and learn.

---

[2]Jeanne Achterberg, *Imagery in Healing* (Boston: Shambhala, 1985), p. 180.

[3]*Ibid.*, p.173.

[4]Neville Hodgkinson, *Will to be Well* (York Beach, Maine: Samuel Weiser, Inc., 1984), p. 9.

[5]Dennis T. Jaffe, Ph.D., *Healing From Within* (New York: Simon & Schuster, Inc., 1986), p. 143.

[6]Hodgkinson, p. 30.

Traditional Chinese medicine has long viewed health in terms of balance in an even larger sense. The individual is seen as a microcosm in the macrocosm, subject to universal laws. Living in disharmony with the "ultimate principle" results in physical or psychological disease; balance and harmony must be re-established in order to produce a lasting cure.[7]

When illness does occur, it is an opportunity to examine ourselves and our circumstances. Illness may indicate that we have gotten out of balance, that we need to be more compassionate with ourselves. When disease develops, it may be a clue that we need some form of adjustment, whether in our external circumstances or in our responses to circumstances. Adjusting the physical environment can aid recovery, whether by removing a source of debilitation or by stimulating self-exploration, activity, and hope.

Many of us in contemporary Western culture feel isolated in the world and carry numerous inner schisms. We rarely notice the seasonal shifts in the sun's course, the phases of the moon, or the signs of a change in the weather. And we've forgotten that these and many other factors still influence our state of being. We have inner voices we don't heed, parts of ourselves we don't love, and psychic depths and heights that go unexplored.

But health derives in large part from a feeling of wholeness—of connection with the multidimensional worlds within and without—a feeling that we make sense, that we have a right to be. Such wholeness encompasses feelings of rootedness, purpose, communication, harmony, vitality, love, and opportunities for expression. Healing the divisions within us and between our "inner" and "outer" worlds unblocks the flow of life energy in and through us. The balanced flow of that energy is the state of vital health.

For nearly every dimension of health, there is a corresponding aspect of our built environment. Disharmonious environments can be sources of physical and mental stress, but our surroundings can

---

[7]David E. Bresler, Ph.D., "Chinese Medicine and Holistic Health," in *Health for the Whole Person*, ed. by Arthur C. Hastings et al. (Boulder, Colorado: Westview Press, 1980), p. 408.

also encourage us to relax, help us to learn about ourselves and our world, encourage self-expression, and reflect to us the best in ourselves. At base, healing environments do two things particularly well: they connect us with vital, positive forces, and they enhance our ability to respond to the anti-life forces we may encounter.

Our personal environment mirrors our world view and our sense of self. It gives us messages about our oneness with, or alienation from, the pulse of life. It can reflect either our magical nature or our boredom and powerlessness. It becomes both an extension and a molder of our most basic drives.

What qualities should we look for in evaluating the healthfulness of an existing place, or as an aid in creating a new environment? I propose that healing environments:

1. stimulate positive awareness of ourselves;
2. enhance our connections with nature, culture, and people;
3. allow for privacy;
4. do us no physical harm;
5. provide meaningful, varying stimuli;
6. encourage times of relaxation;
7. allow us to interact with them productively;
8. balance constancy and flexibility;
9. be beautiful.

I will discuss each item briefly here and expand on these themes throughout the book.

1. *Stimulate positive awareness of ourselves.* As we inhabit and adjust our environment, it becomes a mirror for everything within us. It can be a tool for learning about ourselves, a vehicle for self-expression, and a means for change as we reflect in our environment qualities we like or want to encourage in ourselves. Our environment can be a three-dimensional affirmation of our wholeness and our magical nature. It can increase our awareness of our body, mind, and soul, our past and our potential. It can embody reminders of things that make us happy or give us hope. It can offer us opportunities to explore and to expand ourselves. When we decorate our homes or equip our offices to impress others,

according to the dictates of fashion, we sap our strength by running our lives for others rather than using our environment to strengthen our sense of ourselves.

2. Enhance our connections with nature, culture, and people. We need to feel that we have a place in the world. If we share a home or workplace with others, the nature and arrangement of spaces, materials, lighting, and furniture can stimulate or inhibit interactions among people. If we have a strong ethnic heritage, our buildings can help us feel rooted by reflecting the related aesthetics and traditions. And, wherever we are, any opportunities we have to appreciate the world of nature from indoors can remind us of our belonging in a larger scheme of things. By their very walled nature, buildings are excellent at isolating people from the earth, the sun, seasons, plants and animals, and each other. It takes awareness to reestablish the connections and create buildings that are inclusive and embracing.

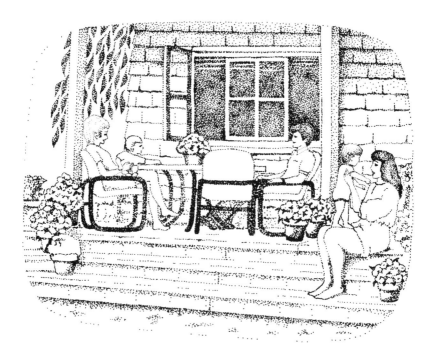

3. Allow for privacy. In Western cultures, privacy is as important to our sense of self as is social interaction. The need for privacy goes hand in hand with the need for a measure of control over our lives. In many workplaces, privacy is the privilege of the upper ranks; lack of it in the lower echelons can diminish one's sense of integrity. Even in the standard home, a couple's "private space" is shared; rarely do partners each have a room to call their own. In privacy we can become acquainted with ourselves, strengthen our identity, and restore inner balance.

4. Do us no physical harm. It seems obvious that we would not want to make buildings that harm our bodies—yet it's being done every day. Toxic materials, stressful lighting, unnerving noise, and unhealthy heating and air conditioning systems can all work against our well-being and are present, to varying degrees, in many contemporary buildings. For some people, simply getting out of range of hazardous building materials and systems will make a marked difference in their health. But we mustn't stop there. Using non-toxic materials, we can still make alienating buildings that sap our vitality and cripple our will.

5. Provide meaningful, varying stimuli. Our organisms are not made for monotony. Our bodies need change to thrive. When we are exposed to unchanging temperature, lighting levels, noise, and sights, and when nothing around us moves or grows, our senses become dull and we function poorly. On the other hand, when our senses are overstimulated, we can lose our acuity; we shut down in self-defense. We need the kind of input that keeps us tuned up and aware of the world around us without assaulting us.

6. Encourage times of relaxation. Peaceful sounds, calming colors, soft lighting, comfortable furniture, simple surroundings, a pleasant vista, and freedom from interruption are great aids to relaxation. Many of us live in high gear, and our primary health need is often simply to relax so that we can restore our vitality. If you work at a high-pressure job, you might want your whole home to encourage relaxation. Better still would be a special room at work and one at home devoted just to relaxing. Simply knowing that we have a place where we can escape to balance ourselves can give us the serenity to get through times of stress. And the more we use one special place for relaxation, the more quickly we become relaxed when we enter it.

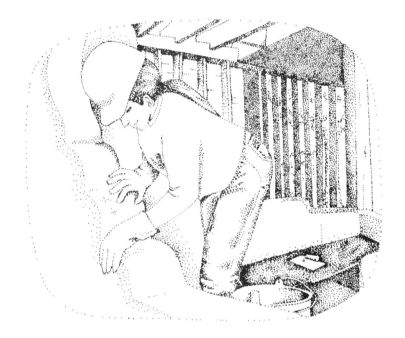

7. *Allow us to interact with them productively.* Our health is influenced by our feelings of self-determination, control, accomplishment, and freedom of expression. What better arena than our immediate surroundings for developing these feelings? Self-determination can mean anything from the ability to open and close a window to suit yourself, to conceiving and executing a remodeling job. Taking responsibility for your environment combats feelings of helplessness. Any way in which you maintain, adjust, or improve your environment in nurturing ways can increase your sense of importance and capability. Any time you imagine and carry out an environmental improvement—no matter how small—you achieve not only a physical result, but also enduring evidence of your ability to change your world for the better. Any time you put something of yourself into your environment, you give yourself a

lasting gift. Such care increases feelings of self-love, and encourages us to be more giving with others.

8. *Contain a balance between constancy and flexibility*. High levels of external challenge and change are often accompanied by internal confusion and disease. Yet illness can also result from too much rigidity or too little challenge. We want freedom and stimulation, but we also want security. In fact, the more secure we feel in certain areas of our lives, the more adaptable to change we are in other areas. The constant aspect of a building could be a structural framework that remains over centuries while alterations can be made to accommodate different uses as time goes by; it could be the use of a traditional architectural style that has meaning to the locale or the dwellers; it could even be a special area rug that accompanies you to each new apartment you rent. Flexibility can come from furniture and partitions that can be rearranged, a structure that is easily added to, an atypical approach to how you inhabit existing spaces, and anything that you use in different positions such as windows, doors, lights, and blinds. Healing environments are able to reflect both changes in the season and changes in the people who inhabit them.

9. *Be beautiful*. The creation and experience of beauty is immediate, whole, and healing. It enlivens our senses, warms our hearts, relaxes us, and puts us at one with the entire surround. The concept of esthetics, by contrast, seems to be superficial, hard-edged, and impersonal; it's more an idea than an experience, and it puts us in the realm of criticism and competition. Beauty appears to arise naturally from a holistic belief system, while ugly buildings and products are easily created in a world where it is deemed possible to separate process from product. Mark Holborn, in his history of Japanese landscape design, offered:

> As soon as the striving for beauty was self-conscious, forced, or pretentious, then beauty was lost. Beauty flourished where there was least desire to create it—in the accidents of Nature. . . . The role of the artist was to act as the agent through which beauty took form, not as a creator or controller extracting beauty.[8]

---

[8]Mark Holborn, *The Ocean in the Sand* (Boulder, Colorado: Shambhala, 1978), p. 19.

As a wise man said long ago, "Love is the essence, and beauty is the manifestation."

Just as health is a dynamic state, so is environmental healing. The entire process of creating and inhabiting a place is as important to our well-being as the place itself. The increased awareness, the acts of caring for oneself, and the sense of meaningful involvement and accomplishment that accompany the undertaking enrich our lives in an upspiralling way.

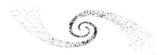

What in your present environment feels healing to you? Notice every object, color, texture, space, and enclosure. Notice the temperature and quality of the air. Listen to the sounds. Where does your environment yield to you and where does it resist you? Where do you go when you want to be alone? When you want to be with others? When you want to work? When you want to relax? When you feel bad? When you are happy? What image of yourself does your environment reflect to you?

Imagine that your environment helps you to feel in touch with yourself, peaceful, and connected with the pulse of life; what is it like?

· CHAPTER · 3 ·

Indoors, Outdoors

*We tend to forget our connection to the earth, to the sky,
to each other, to the life that's constantly percolating in and around us.
When we forget our connections, we wind up feeling drained and
isolated. When we remember our connections, we become energized, inspired, and feel a part of all that's around us.*

—MARGO ADAIR

As a species, we have evolved through millenia of direct interaction with sun, wind, rain, soil, fire, plants, and animals in daily and seasonal cycles. We are members of a complex matrix of self-regulating systems. Our basic physiological requirements, anatomical structures, and psychological drives have not changed much since the Stone Age, and—barring genetic tinkering—are not likely to change for many generations to come.

As individuals, our first home was a human body. It kept us warm, rocked us in amniotic juices, nourished us through the navel, and surrounded us with the sound of a heartbeat. Through our mother's biological rhythms, we were keyed to the cycles of days and seasons. Subconsciously, we often long to return to that soft, secure, living world we once knew.

With this rich biological heritage, we now sit in our houses, schools, and workplaces, breathing tainted recycled air, receiving impoverished or artificial solar radiation, hearing the droning of machines, missing the triggers to our biological clocks, and alternately understimulating and overstimulating our senses. Our buildings rarely give us useful information or remind us of our place in the fabric of life; instead they tell us that we are small and powerless.

The triumph of modern living has been to seal us off from the outside world and create an indoor world that we can modify at will. We have made buildings into extensions of our bodies—tools of evolution that allow us to "adapt" to an immense range of climates. This puts us into an intimate survival relationship with our buildings, yet they create an impoverished milieu com-

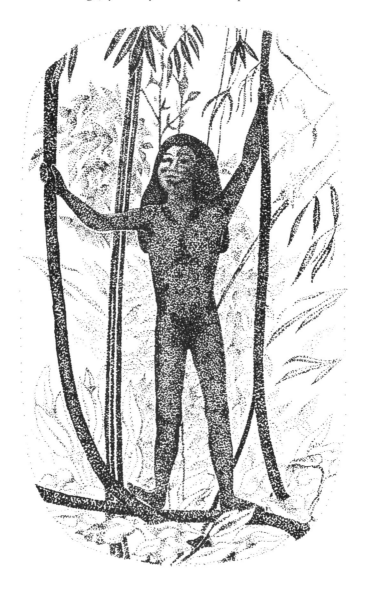

pared to the environment for which we are genetically adapted. It is a paradox: we make buildings to keep us warm, dry, and organized so that we can flourish, yet those very buildings often stand in the way of our flourishing. Biologist Rene Dubos notes that "the factories and offices we have created to help relieve us of the stress of surviving are promoting an unprecedented number of stress-related illnesses; . . . the technologies we have created to cure disease and prolong life are causing new diseases and perpetuating lives that lack vitality."[1]

When we left the cave and the open country, we may have also left behind things we still need. Nobody knows how many of our internal processes are triggered by environmental clues that are missing or distorted when we are indoors. Only in recent decades have we learned that much of our biochemistry relies on sunlight, and that many of our internal rhythms are regulated by external cycles, some of which are masked inside of buildings. Even our mental alertness relies on the stimulation of a varied, changing surrounding that is rich with meaningful information. This is not to say that the noble savage enjoyed perfect health, but it does suggest that we are missing something when we deny ourselves conditions to which we are best adapted.

The truth of this came home to me several years ago. I was living in a Berkeley studio apartment and apprenticing in an architecture office. I was always busy, tired, and out of sync, and I dealt with the world through my mind. Needing a break, I went to Big Sur, on the California coast, for a few days. At first I frustrated myself; whenever I arrived somewhere, I tried to jump up and rush off to someplace else. Eventually something inside said, "Just sit there. Don't get up, don't do anything, don't think about it, just sit there." I think I was afraid I'd be bored. Gradually, as my mind quieted down, I began to notice things. I was sitting on the bank of the Big Sur River. The water was clear and shallow, and I became aware that the stones of the riverbed were beautiful. I gazed at them through the moving water, noticing the subtle ripples they caused. Then I noticed the sounds—the soft, steady rushing of the water, the calls of birds, the footfall of small animals. And the smells—the freshness of water, the pungency of

---

[1] Rene Dubos in Hastings, *Health for the Whole Person*, p. 12.

trees, the richness of earth. I noticed that my whole skin could feel the ambience—that with my eyes closed I could tell where the river was by the cool, moist air, and where the sun was by the radiant warmth. I lost track of time. I was a part of everything.

I spent days at Big Sur in that state of surrender. I occasionally moved from one place to another just to experience a different range of sensations. I was open. I felt clear, whole, and healthy. The birds, the trees, the sun, the water, the rocks, the breezes, and the plants were all teaching me. All I had to do was Be.

As I returned to Berkeley, I vowed not to shut down again. I would keep my senses alive, I would take time to be still, to receive and learn. When I got to my apartment, I lay on my back on the floor. It was hard and flat and cold. I saw around me furniture, white walls, and a white ceiling. Nothing moved. The indirect sunlight from the windows told me nothing. My ears were open: the refrigerator came on, a radio blared, a car chugged up the street. There was no texture, no enriching variation, no useful information. I understood why I had shut down and lived in my mind. I began to wonder if such an extreme contrast between Big Sur and my apartment was necessary; I knew it wasn't healthy.

No building will ever be a substitute for those wild places. But neither would we choose to give up living in buildings for very long. We create our shelters in response to a range of physiological, psychological, and spiritual needs. Altering the environment is as natural to life as eating, sleeping, and procreating; organisms at all levels transform their surroundings and, reciprocally, adapt to the new conditions they have created. Buildings have a valid role as mediators between ourselves and an "outside world" that is not always safe or comfortable. But it's unnecessary—even deadly—for our indoor environments to be as impoverished as they are.

Perhaps the problem begins in our minds, when we perceive ourselves as separate from nature. Indoor austerity arises from a world view that says it is possible to separate one thing from another, and that we can do so without repercussion. But in fact we are an integral part of nature. We need the nourishment and stimulation of the living whole.

We can revive the built environment by studying the untamed world. We can bring plants and animals indoors, recreating a living milieu under conditions comfortable to us. We can observe the structure of nature and apply its lessons to the design of indoor spaces, creating diversity, richness, and stimulation around us.

We can also increase the physical connections between indoors and outdoors. The traditional Japanese home had large openings that provided good ventilation and broad views of gardens. While this exposed dwellers to temperature extremes, architect Yuichiro Kodama says, "The Japanese people found pleasure in the seasonal variations that dictated the rhythm of life. . . . This kind of thinking has taught the Japanese to confirm and coexist with nature rather than to go against it.[2]" Kodama believes that in modern air-conditioned buildings this sensibility has been replaced by boredom.

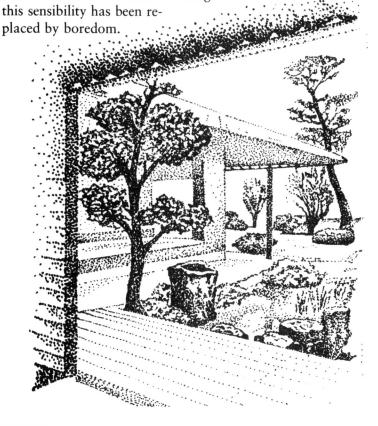

---

[2]Yuichiro Kodama, "A House for All Seasons" (paper presented at the Environmental Evolution and Technologies Conference, University of Texas at Austin, August, 1975).

We don't have to choose either extreme. We can design places that encourage us to eat, sleep, or socialize outdoors in favorable weather, returning indoors when we prefer. We can have whole walls that roll aside, opening our indoors to the outdoors. We can create semi-enclosed spaces that modify climate but keep us in touch with fresh air, sounds, and sights.

We do not need to give up indoor living but rather to transform it. We need to learn what sorts of contact with the untamed world are important to our vitality. We need to explore how a holistic world view plays out in the buildings we create. We must heed the inner clues that tell us what we need more of and what we need less of. Rather than drawing rigid boundaries, we can achieve healthful flow and mediation between "indoors" and "outdoors."

Our evolution and our adaptation to the environments we alter is a recurring theme throughout this book. Our genetic and cultural heritage is an indispensable touchstone. Rene Dubos once said, ". . . in an ever-changing world each period and each type of civilization will continue to have its burden of diseases created by the unavoidable failures of adaptation to the new environment."[3] We can minimize those failures if we base our choices on knowledge of our own nature.

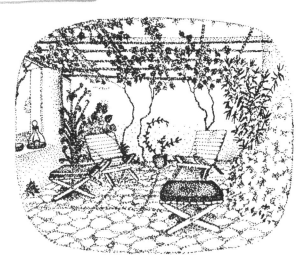

---

[3]Dubos, Rene, *Man Adapting* (New Haven: Yale University Press, 1965), p. 346.

CHAPTER 4

Awareness
and Empowerment

Connectedness . . . may very well be the ability
of the individual to be in touch with the environment with all
the senses and with all aspects of primitive experience.
—LEONARD DUHL, M.D.

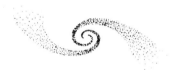

Pause a moment where you are now. Feel the chair that is holding
you. Take a deep breath and relax. Notice how the air feels on
your skin: is it warm, cool, still, moving, dry, humid? What
sounds can you hear, indoors and out? Notice the steady back-
ground sounds as well as the intermittent ones. What do the
sounds tell you about your world? What can you smell? Let your
eyes go out of focus and see your world as light, color, and shapes.
What do you see? As you refocus your eyes, where are they drawn?
What do you see around you that pleases you? What do you see
that makes you uncomfortable? How spacious or enclosed is the
area? How does the place feel to you?

Try this again in different places—ones that feel good, ones
that feel bad, ones where you spend most of your time. You'll
begin to notice patterns that can serve as tools for you.

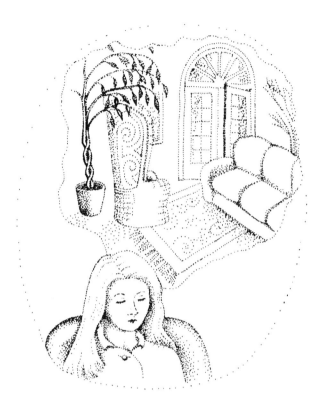

In primitive societies, such environmental awareness has had a high survival value. Self-observation, identification, testing, exploration, memory of sights and routes, awareness of ecosystems and seasons, cooperation, and reliance on instincts are an integral part of life. By contrast, our Western culture seems to value numbness. We may fear that if we become more sensitive we will only feel more pain: we'll realize that the food has no flavor, the air smells funny, the fluorescent lights buzz, the city looks tawdry, we're lonely, our head aches, and we just don't care. We've forgotten how good being alive can feel.

When we let distant authorities and social pressures set the standards for our thoughts and actions, we don't observe for ourselves what's going on or how we really feel about things. When decisions that affect our lives and habitats are made by people we never see, we lack a sense of participation and influence. We become exhausted from living out of sync with ourselves, and we can no longer tell how our environment is affecting us. We tell ourselves that any adverse effects are either inconsequential or unavoidable and that we must be doing okay because we're getting by somehow. This shut-down state produces apathy and alienation, increasing our susceptibility to disease.

The antidote to this state is awareness. Without awareness we are powerless; with awareness we need never feel bored or cut off. When we heighten our sensitivity to the worlds within and around us, we begin the process of self-healing and empowerment. Awareness without a sense of personal power or the tools to initiate change could indeed be frustrating. But the message here is that you can transform things. By increasing your awareness, you will not make things any worse than they are, but only through awareness can you begin to make things better.

The simple act of choosing to pay attention to your world sends positive, healing messages to your self: I deserve good care, I can change my surroundings for the better, I know best what feels good to me. Once you begin to feel hopeful, you'll know that you can get past the pain of being aware in a stressful world, and into the joy of improving your situation. The subsequent steps of acquiring useful knowledge and taking action can carry you further on an upspiral of vitality.

Awareness takes slowing down, relaxing, quieting the buzz in our heads, and letting ourselves listen, look, and feel. The messages we get from within and around us are rarely linear and logical; they're complex and multi-level. A place has myriad qualities, yet it is a whole. As you learn to tune into the parts and the whole, you will better understand what gives different places their unique qualities.

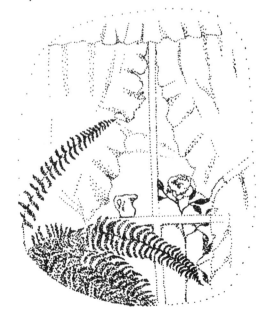

Awareness isn't just the first of a series of steps; it is an on-going state that is the core of healing yourself and your environments. You are a sensitive receiver who can observe, intuit, and synthesize what no one else can. Your continuing awareness will lead you to react to existing conditions in new ways, conceive of uniquely appropriate changes for your environment, and select the right tools, materials, and means to do the job. As you stay attuned to your evolving environment, you can make adjustments and respond to unanticipated opportunities. Your awareness may not spring forth full blown, and the changes you want to make around you will take time, but the point is to start where you are.

Throughout the process of learning about health and environment, keep listening to your inner voice. Someone might tell you that a particular climate, house shape, color scheme, or light fixture will be healthy for you, but you're the one who will be living with them. All the theory in the world won't make them work if they don't feel good to you. Do look beyond yourself for inspiration and education, but don't sell out your perceptions. Even ancient wisdom about the design and placement of buildings can be lifeless when applied by rote, divorced from the spark that created it. That spark lives today—in you.

It's as easy to get caught up in the physical aspects of the environment as it is to concentrate on the physical component of human health. Toxic materials, dead air, poor light, and noise are all real. But we also need to go deeper—to get beyond the "symptom level." As a culture we wouldn't be producing these unhealthy environments if we weren't cut off from ourselves, from feedback, and from the joy of life. And as individuals, we will not touch our deeper, health-affecting malaise just by changing light fixtures, nor will we reach the vibrant joy in life that is possible by simply altering our environment out of context with the real meaning of our lives.

In fact, inner and outer awareness could be the most effective tool you have for changing your surroundings. How you feel about yourself and what you are open to around you form the basis for how you experience a place. Just as we sometimes project our mental state onto other people, missing what they might have to offer us, so do we tend to see our milieu through the filter of our personality, moods, and experiences. The same place can feel hostile or loving, with the only change being in ourselves. We see around us that which mirrors our inner landscape. If you want to be in a place you love, start by loving yourself and life. Look around you for things you love, even if there is only one small thing. It might be a plant, a color, the way the light falls on the floor, a person, or a favorite curio. See how many things or qualities you can find that evoke warmth or delight in you. By becom-

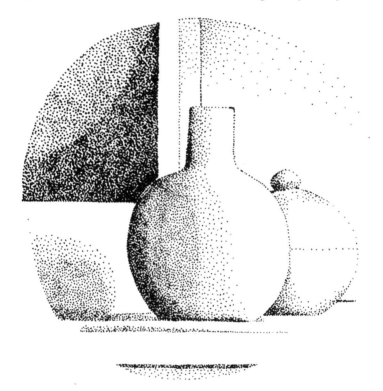

ing aware of yourself and the wonder inside you, you begin to resonate with what is wonderful around you. And pretty soon your world looks different.

I learned that lesson one dreary winter. I was often sick, wasn't making much money, and hated the oppressive house I lived in. I wanted to move, but I felt resourceless. A friend lent me an inspiring book, and I curled up in bed to read it. Losing myself in the story lifted me out of my misery and restored my sense of the rightness of things, the love in myself, and a broader perspective on life. When I looked up from the book, I was surprised to notice that my whole house seemed different. Everything about it felt good; I felt fortunate to be living there. I noticed appealing features that I had overlooked in my earlier grumblings. The house was reflecting my renewed love of life.

A friend of mine found another way to change his environment via his perceptions. His heart was in the Sierras, but his work was in San Francisco. He made his peace with the city by knowing the origins of its parts: the granite veneer on his high-rise office building was quarried in the mountains; his drinking water came from the snowfall of the Sierra Nevada; his Victorian row-house was built from the redwood forests; the sun that shone on him also shone on the ocean, the Bay, the Delta, the Central Valley, and the Sierras. He simply chose to see things around him in a way that linked him with the things he loved.

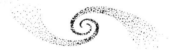

Find a quiet spot, make yourself comfortable, and relax. Imagine that you are in an indoor place where you are at peace, radiant, and healthy. You can have anything that feels good to you in this place; there are no limitations. Notice what is below your feet: the textures, materials, colors, warmth, or coolness. Notice how the air feels, the sounds you hear, the scents you smell. See what is in front of you, on either side of you, behind you, above you. In your imagination, walk around this place, feeling the textures, seeing the light and the colors, noticing how every detail contributes to the overall good feeling. Be aware of any furniture, art, plants, animals, artifacts, rugs, or toys.

Now be aware of how this place connects to the outside. Are there walls, windows, doors? What are they like?

Walk outside, where the surroundings are also attuned to you. Notice what is around you, how the air feels and smells, what sounds you hear. Look at the landscape—plants, water, earth, sky, animals, structures, surfaces, fences, outdoor furniture. Notice how other people and the rest of the world come into this picture.

How do you feel in this place? Keep that feeling as you return to where you are now.

The place where you have just been is within you and is always available to you. Look for things around you—big or little—that resonate with your imaginary healing place. Know that you can begin to change the parts of your current environment that aren't harmonious. As you move through this book, you will focus on different aspects of your surroundings. As your awareness grows, you can continue to make changes to bring this vision and reality together.

· CHAPTER · 5 ·

Self Knowledge,
Home, and the Heart

*Nothing is easier to see than consciousness once we recognize
that it is embodied in the forms and structures we create.*
—STARHAWK

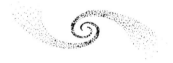

*Take a few moments to relax and recall your earliest childhood
impressions of the world around you. It might take a while, but
just let your mind drift backward in time until the images become
clearer.*

*In your memories, which senses stand out? Do you recall the
smells, the people around you, colors? Are there strong emotions
associated with any environments: feeling contented in the sunlight, scared and isolated in a closed room, important in your high
chair at the table? If you don't have much recollection of your
childhood, fantasize yourself as a child in different environments
and imagine your gut reactions. Relax and let your mind roam;
such fantasies and memories will evoke some of your most basic
impressions and values. Don't try too hard to interpret them. Just
notice your reactions, and notice any insights that come to you
about how these memories relate to the present. Sometimes early
impressions express basic drives or preferences that form who we*

are; if listened to, they can increase our enjoyment of life. But sometimes they are prejudices that come from associating a particular event with its surroundings, causing us unconsciously to limit ourselves in adulthood.

Now recall the home where you grew up. If there were several, choose the one that means the most to you. Notice where you are in the house in your first image: in the living room, your bedroom, the kitchen, the yard? Move through the house, recalling the shapes and sizes of the rooms, memorable events that took place there, the people you lived with, the furnishings, the windows, the lighting, sounds, smells, the feel of each room, and any details that come to mind. What are the surfaces like? Does the house feel warm, cool, sunny, shadowy? What sounds can you hear? What can you see through the windows? Are there rooms or places where you feel welcome, and rooms that are off limits? Are there scary places, intriguing places? Do you have a favorite spot? Who else lives in the house, and which rooms are their territories?

Now go outside the house. Is there a yard, a city street, open fields? Is there a place for you? How do you feel about the area around your house? How does it relate to the rest of the vicinity— other homes, streets, the city, town or countryside?

You may find it helpful to make a drawing of this home. It needn't be technically accurate; what's important is that it embody

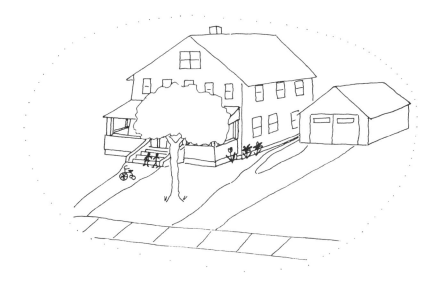

your impressions. Use sketches, floor plans, words, symbols, colors, and whatever else will help you perceive the ways in which you related to that home. You might even want to do this exercise with a friend, and describe your childhood homes to each other after exploring them in your minds; in expressing something to someone else, we often have insights that might not have come otherwise.

Are any features of your childhood home reflected in your current preferences and attitudes? Don't look just at the physical aspects, but also be aware of what you learned early in life about "inner" and "outer." As a child, what did you experience about the continuity or separation between you and the world around you? How did you perceive the difference between your home and the world beyond?

These explorations are valuable whether you are creating a healing environment alone or with others. Expressing your own preferences will help you feel like an important part of a shared environment; discussing these exercises with others will deepen your connections to each other and your sensitivity to others in general; seeking the images that the group has in common and finding places for individual expression will establish a rich base for all your activities together. If you are creating a place where others will come (an office, a healing center, a school), these and other exercises in the book will help you become aware of qualities that may be universally welcoming, peaceful, and evocative. They will also reveal your idiosyncrasies so that you can avoid imposing them on others.

As infants grow, they move from perceiving their mothers as the whole environment to becoming aware of other people and their surroundings. "The house becomes [the child's] world, its very cosmos. From being a shadowy shell glimpsed out of half-closed eyes, the house becomes familiar, recognized, a place of security and love."[1] As perceptions increase, a child's world becomes divided into "home" and "everything else." Later, as the

---

[1]Clare Cooper, "The House as Symbol of the Self," in Lang, John, ed., *Designing for Human Behavior* (Stroudsburg, Pennsylvania: Dowden, Hutchinson, & Ross, Inc., 1974), p. 138.

child approaches adulthood and establishes a working relationship with the world beyond, home retains special meaning as a place of security and roots—a symbol of self, family, and love.

As adults, home is still the place where we spend most of our time, and the environment over which we have the greatest control. Home becomes an extension of the self and a metaphor for the body. Our homes express our beliefs about the distinction between self and the rest of the world: physically, the boundaries of our dwellings enclose a microclimate which we adjust for our comfort; psychologically and symbolically those boundaries take on further meaning. The walls of our house represent the power to admit or exclude—to choose which people, sights, sounds, and elements we want to have around us. In our homes, we can surround ourselves with familiar and pleasing things; we can relax and let down our guard. We can establish order in a world that may otherwise seem chaotic or out of our control. According to environmental analyst Clare Cooper Marcus, people for whom the world is dangerous and hostile are likely to place greater emphasis on the house as a fortress or retreat, while people who feel less threatened are more likely to regard the home as a place for self-expression and enjoyment of self or family.[2]

Within the home, our environment expresses our relationship with ourselves. If we feel weak or inconsequential, we may be passive, accepting the place as it is or leaving its creation to others; we put up with inconvenience, shut down the unencouraged parts of ourselves, and do all the molding and adapting inside. The inner tension and alienation produced can express themselves in a variety of ills. In contrast, when we feel sure of our right to be, we treat our environment as a friend, a partner, a place to express and explore ourselves. Carl G. Jung said of his home: "I am in the midst of my true life, I am most deeply myself."[3]

Our interactions with our surroundings are a source of continuous feedback. Consciously and unconsciously, expressing ourselves in our environment lets us see who we are and helps us shape who we become. Our choices and arrangements of furni-

---

[2]*Ibid.*, p. 134.
[3]Carl G. Jung, *Memories, Dreams, Reflections* (London: Collins, The Fontana Library Series, 1969), p. 253, as quoted in Cooper, p. 140.

ture, the things we put on the walls, the music we play, the colors we select, and the ways we use each room all give us messages, reinforcing our beliefs about ourselves.

On a rudimentary level, my own home quickly reflects whether I am taking good care of myself. When I am so busy that I forget to treat myself lovingly, I see dirty dishes, unopened mail, dying houseplants, and films of dust; I soon become both inconvenienced and disheartened. But when I begin to care for myself, my environment soon becomes more ordered and joyous; the flourishing houseplant returns the love I give it, clean dishes are available when I need them, and I see around me evidence of my capabilities and creativity, all of which help me feel more confident. This feedback loop can be entered at any point: when I start to care for my environment, I start to feel better about myself; when I feel good about myself, I interact positively with my environment.

A dynamic, loving relationship with your surroundings can be a constant source of vitality and hope—qualities that create the will to thrive at the cellular level. Having a home where you feel secure, self-aware, expressive, and connected with life plays a great role in your health and well-being. In her book, *Home-Psych,* Joan Kron says,

> Multiple acts of personalization that aren't any more world-shaking than figuring out where to hang a picture, deciding how many plants to put on the windowsill, selecting which vegetables to grow in the garden, or choosing the sheet pattern add up to a sense of competence and control. . . . To be surrounded by things we have chosen ourselves gives us a sense of security.[4]

A connection with the past is a major psychological component of environmental comfort. Cooper Marcus has found that people's images of their ideal environments often bear a remarkable resemblance to the ones in which they grew up.[5] Symbolic ties with one's younger self, one's family, and one's culture bestow a sense of belonging, of having a rightful place in the continuity of life. As philosopher Mircea Eliade wrote, "Habitations are not

---

[4]Joan Kron, *Home-Psych* (New York: Clarkson N. Potter, Inc., Publishers, 1983), p. 56.
[5]Cooper, p. 145.

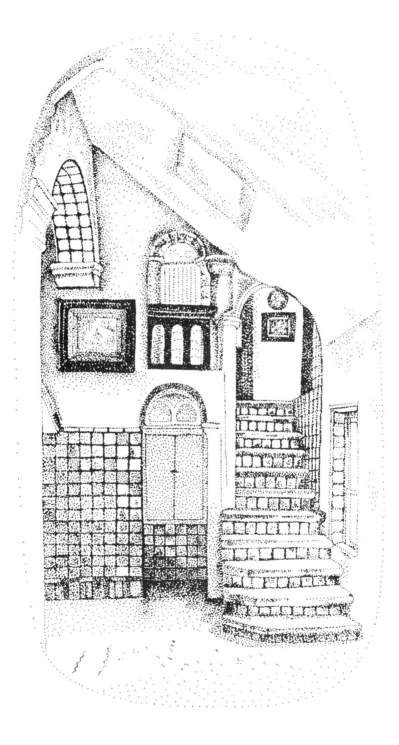

lightly changed, for it is not easy to abandon one's world."[6]

Though we can gain strength from acknowledging our roots, we may also need a feeling of freedom and a sense that we are special in place and time. We need to know that, while we have a past, we are neither confined nor defined by it. Designer Catherine C. Crane says, "It's not a comfortable feeling to believe you could be anybody. It's better to be in an environment that supports your uniqueness, that builds on and enhances your interests . . ."[7]

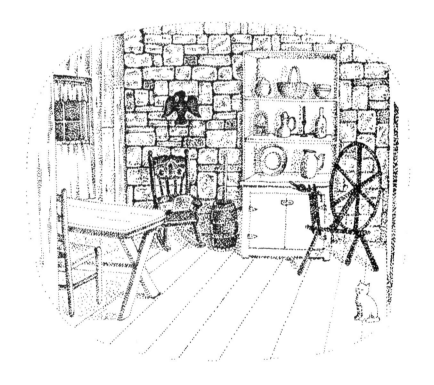

---

[6]Mircea Eliade, *The Sacred and the Profane* (New York: Harcourt, 1959) pp. 56-57, quoted in Cooper, p. 143.

[7]Catherine C. Crane, *Personal Places* (New York: Whitney Library of Design, 1982), p. 122.

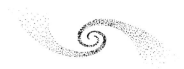

What does your present home say to you about who you are? About how you relate to yourself? About how you relate to the outside world? How nurturing is your home to you? Does the place seem to express you? Does it confine you? What has motivated the choices you've made about your home environment? Does your home help you feel continuity with your past? Which parts of your home receive most of your attention? Which parts do you neglect? Does anything in your home encourage you to grow and express yourself?

As you explore your inner landscape and its outward projections, you will be healing both yourself and your world. That sense of integration—of the power to perceive, nurture, and actualize—can bring increasing harmony and wholeness.

> There is one environment
> That stands above all.
> It is the environment
> That lives in your spirit.
> Nourish it well.
> And all else follows in time.
>
> —TOM BENDER

· II ·
A·S·P·E·C·T·S ·O·F·
·H·E·A·L·I·N·G·
E·N·V·I·R·O·N·M·E·N·T·S·

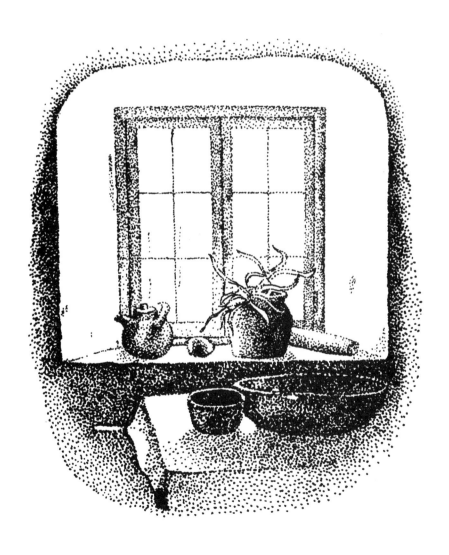

· CHAPTER · 6 ·

Symbols and
Environmental Messages

*In many societies outside the West, symbols and
symbolic actions are essential ingredients of human understanding of,
and relationships with, reality, including relationships with
the human as well as the sacred. In the West, it is increasingly
suggested that a lack of adequate symbolism
is part of the modern malaise.*

—RICHARD CAVENDISH

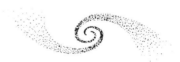

*Choose an object that you can look at right now. Does simply
looking at it evoke any response in you? Where did this object
come from? What associations do you have with its past? What
does this object say about you to others? What does its appearance
say about its place in time: is it high-tech, early American, primitive, timeless? Does it carry a sense of a particular country or
region? What size and form does it have in relation to you, and
in relation to its surroundings? What messages does that give you?
How do you respond to its color? Is the object useful? Decorative?
Notice the materials, texture, sound, and smell; do they evoke any
thoughts or feelings?*

By now you have probably learned things you'd barely sus-
pected about the meanings that one object can have for you. You
have learned more about yourself and your values, as well as about
how many ways you can be connected to (or alienated from) some-
thing.

Now look around the room. Notice the relationships among
the different aspects of the room—objects, surfaces, forms, spaces,
lighting, and so on. What are the largest objects in the room? The
smallest? The brightest? Notice how things are grouped or juxta-
posed. What messages do you get from the place as a whole? What
does this environment say about you to yourself? To others?

A symbol is anything that represents something else, that implies things greater or other than itself. Every aspect of your environment carries symbolic meaning, and these symbols affect you
whether or not you're conscious of them. Because of the intimate
connections between sensory inputs, mental reactions, and physiological functioning, your whole system is constantly responding
to symbolism. The symbols around you may trigger relaxation,
apprehension, hope, distrust, and so on. When the "real" and the
"symbolic" disagree, we often respond more strongly to the symbolic. Pavlov demonstrated this when he trained dogs to salivate
at the sound of a bell; to the dogs, the bell "meant" food. Biologist Rene Dubos refers to "[man's] propensity to symbolize everything that happens to him, and then to react to the symbols as if
they were actual environmental stimuli."[1]

Used consciously, symbolism can be a powerful force to aid
your healing and growth by externalizing your desires, feeding
them back to you, and bringing you into alignment with them.
You may currently be subject to conflicting environmental messages or to symbolic information that undermines your well-being.
But by choosing symbols that reflect the best in you, and by minimizing those that decrease your vitality, you can actually contribute to your health.

Symbols act on our inner consciousness, reaching us more
deeply and powerfully—and often more subtly—than reasoned ar-

---

[1]Rene Dubos, *Man Adapting* (New Haven, Yale University Press, 1965), p. 7.

guments. Furthermore, they often embody relationships or connections that we miss when thinking linearly, directly evoking a sense of wholeness.

> The great function of symbols is to point beyond themselves, in the power of that to which they point, to open up levels of reality which otherwise are closed, and to open up levels of the human mind of which we are otherwise not aware.[2]

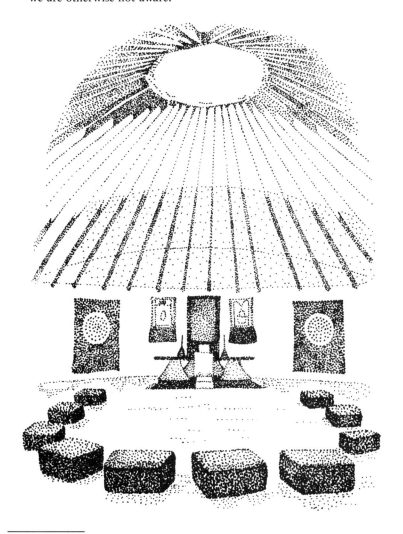

[2]Paul Tillich in *Man, Myth, and Magic*, ed. by Richard Cavendish (New York: Marshall Cavendish Corporation, 1970), p. 2755.

The time-honored symbolism of the moon "links together the moon's changing cycle in the sky, the rhythms and cycles of life on earth, woman, the waters, death and rebirth, and human destiny."[3] The circle, often lacking in modern environments, symbolizes wholeness, the center, and cyclic phenomena; it represents both the infinite and the finite, the boundless and the bounded, completeness and separateness.

Some symbols are highly personal, some have certain meanings within a cultural group, and others are universal. Symbolic

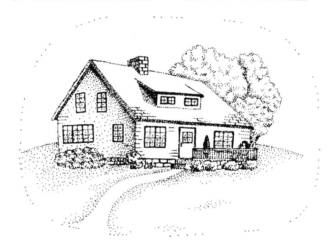

meaning can be acquired by association; the scent of lavender perfume may mean "grandma" to you, or a souvenir may symbolize an event or place. Some items are symbols due to analogous appearance; gold symbolizes the sun, and wavy lines stand for water and flow. Other things have meaning because of their mode of action; the moon symbolizes periodicity, tools symbolize work. Symbolism exists not only in objects but in other qualities such as sequence, motion, sound, and relative position and scale.

> The directions of east, west, north, and south have their own symbolism, as do left and right, and up and down are naturally connected with ideas of progress and decline, superiority and inferiority, good and evil, heaven in the sky and hell underground.[4]

[3] Mircea Eliade in Cavendish, p. 2758.
[4] Cavendish, p. 2758.

Even thermal conditions can be symbolic: a cold room might feel like loneliness and lack of love; a warm greenhouse might evoke memories of a happy summer vacation.

An "environmental message" is the aggregate impression that a building or place gives you; it is what that place tells you about who you are and how you fit into the scheme of things. The popular interest in "human scale" is a reaction against imposing, inhumane buildings that allow us no participation or positive reflection of ourselves. Banks, government buildings, churches, health institutions, and schools have long given us messages that we are small, powerless creatures. By contrast, the detached home with a yard, which most people value highly, tells us that we have autonomy, roots, and a piece of the world to make over in our own image.

In different places, notice what messages the environment is giving you. Watch your body reactions for clues. It may not come easily at first, or you may be overwhelmed by the multiplicity of messages, but as you identify these subliminal inputs, they will lose their power to control you. You can consciously provide an antidote for the negative ones and use the power of positive ones to enhance your life.

Cristina Ismael beautifully described her growing awareness of environmental message content:

> . . . after several days in Mexico City I became aware that I was experiencing something I had felt in many European cities—it did not have to do with similarities in architecture or landscape. Though I couldn't identify it, the feeling kept coming over me in waves. . . .
>
> As the days passed I began to realize that the sensation was linked with the experience of beauty. Parks and gardens everywhere, exquisitely tiled floors and walls, quiet courtyards where lush plants grew, graceful stairwells, statues and fountains, buildings that were centuries old and pleasing because of their age—all this made Mexico City beautiful in the way I had found many European cities beautiful. But knowing this did not help me solve the mystery of the deep stirring I felt walking through the city—a sense that I was different in this environment, as I had been different in Europe.
>
> One afternoon we drove to a small town just south of Mexico City. We arrived near twilight, and stopped to walk around the plaza, in which there were three churches. I was drawn to the largest of these . . . . [A]s I walked through the door my gaze was immediately drawn to the altar, and I realized that the few artifacts of the church had been deliberately and sensitively designed.

In concept and execution, the altar was so pure and light that it looked as if it had been lifted out of the twenty-fifth century and then had been placed, gently and without effort, in the midst of this cathedral silence. The altar was more a statement than a place—a statement made with a few simple, elegant strokes. The highly ornamental sacramental lamps I was used to seeing above the altar in Catholic churches, usually hung from heavy chains, were here represented by graceful ovals of polished brass, which held spheres of red glass in which candles flickered quietly. The cords which held these lamps were nearly invisible, so that at first glance the lamps seemed to be suspended in space. Above the unadorned altar there was a tall, narrow cross of dark wood. Again, there was no detail. It even lacked the traditional figure of Christ. The futuristic design of the altar seemed diametrically opposed to the ancient edifice which housed it, yet they complemented each other perfectly, for they were held together by a theme of stark simplicity and beauty. The building gave this effect by its crudity and immense stone weight, while the altar achieved the same effect with a lightness that was almost ephemeral, and a sophistication of design that seemed beyond our time.

The sensation that I had been experiencing in the city was, in this

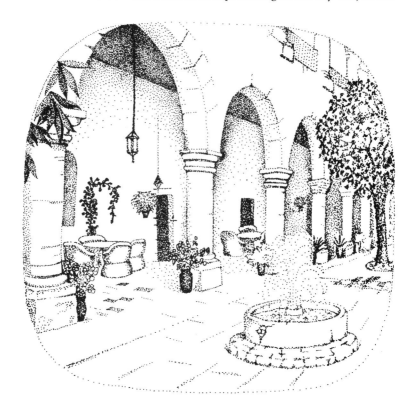

place, so strong that I felt overwhelmed by it. I had to know what I was feeling. I began to walk around the church, listening closely to what was inside, determined to stay in this cathedral until the mystery was solved. After walking in this way for a while I realized that I felt bigger here. Though the size of the building should have emphasized my littleness, I felt instead that I was taller, somehow more expansive in both body and spirit. Then all at once one word struck me with such tremendous force that it felt like an inner explosion: dignity. It was a sense of dignity that I felt in this place, that I felt walking through the streets of Mexico City, that I remembered with longing when I thought of Europe.

For the first time, I saw clearly the incredible effect and impact of environment. In that moment, standing alone in the aisle of that church, I understood that people can be made to feel degenerate or divine by the mere fact of their physical environment. I saw everything around me as a reflection, and understood that we feel ourselves to be what our mirrors tell us we are.[5]

As you become more sensitive to symbolism and environmental messages, you can eliminate or downplay the things around you that symbolize failure, isolation, or powerlessness, and emphasize symbols of capability, happiness, and the continuity of life. Allow your surroundings to be a mirror of the best in you; your vitality will probably increase from that alone. Make your environment symbolize your participation in the rhythms of nature, and alienation is less likely to plague you. Display symbols of your ethnic heritage or your childhood home to give you a sense of roots and continuity.

Become acquainted with your personal symbology. For example, what things or qualities mean love to you: colors, shapes, textures, smells, sounds, volumes? What connotes security? Peacefulness? Order? Connections with nature? What implies tension? Loneliness? Futility?

List the healing qualities you want in your life, and then think about what symbols you associate with each one. Think especially in terms of positive self-awareness, relaxation, productive interaction, familiarity, flexibility, privacy, and connections with nature, culture, and other people.

If you realize that connection with the earth is meaningful to you, you might want earth materials around you—a stone floor,

---

[5]Cristina Ismael, *The Healing Environment* (Millbrae: Celestial Arts, 1976), pp. 16-19.

clay tiles, a brick hearth, or terra cotta flower pots. If you feel like you're in a rut, you could choose symbols of motion and open-ness—more light, active colors, moving water, or whatever is meaningful to you. If you want to make a special place for relax-ation, you might eliminate symbols of mental stimulation, physical activity, or confusion, such as newspapers, bright colors, sports equipment, or clutter; surround yourself instead with symbols of peace and tranquility—calming colors, water, peaceful music, and a few beautiful objects.

Each person has a unique set of symbolic associations. This becomes important when you share a place with other people. A couple I know were in recurring conflict because clutter meant freedom to him, while order meant caring to her. Sometimes rec-ognizing the source of a symbolic difference can suggest a solution and produce greater harmony.

If you are creating a healing place for other people, whether it is a massage studio or a whole health center, look closely at symbol and message content as they might affect others. A mas-seur I know is careful to keep his studio "symbol neutral"; he uses relaxing colors and soft lighting, but avoids anything that might alienate a client such as symbols of specific religions or even "New Age" items like crystals and candles. In such a setting, it is impor-tant to emphasize universal symbols of welcome, nurturing, and calm.

Many people have decried the paucity of symbolism in con-temporary life, but the problem is not a lack of symbols. Rather, it is an abundance of things that symbolize depersonalization, fragmentation, and competition. We don't necessarily need more symbols; we need to be able to read the symbols around us, and we need symbols of continuity, wholeness, community, and self worth. We may live in a fragmented, depersonalized society, but beyond that we are still inhabitants of a beautiful planet in an awe-inspiring solar system, capable of love for ourselves and each other, moved by desires for nourishment, self-expression, and community. Through symbolism, we can stay in touch with our wonderfulness.

· CHAPTER · 7 ·

Light

Where the sun does not enter, the doctor does.
—ITALIAN PROVERB

Without the light of the sun, there would be no life as we know it. Without light and color, our visual world would not exist. Without our inner light, there would be no striving.

Most creation myths involve darkness and light. In some, light is born out of darkness, in others darkness from light, and in others they coexisted from the beginning. But their primacy is universal. Light symbolizes goodness, warmth, activity, creativity, clarity of thought, and spiritual progress, while darkness represents fear, the unknown, coldness, inactivity, unclear perceptions, and unholiness. Yet each has its other side: light is scorching, searing, and dry; darkness is protective, intimate, warm, and fundamental.

> Among the first experiences of a baby must presumably be the sensation of coming out of darkness into light, and all our lives long one of the fixed characteristics of our environment is the alternation of light and darkness, on which we pattern the basic rhythm of our lives.[1]

The therapeutic value of sunlight has been recognized for thousands of years. The Assyrians, Babylonians, and Egyptians all practiced sunbathing for health,[2] and Pliny believed that the pow-

---

[1]Cavendish, *Man, Myth, and Magic,* p. 1622.
[2]Faber Birren, *Light, Color, and Environment* (New York: Van Nostrand Reinhold Company, 1982), p. 14.

er of the Roman Empire stemmed from the fact that Romans took frequent sun- and air-baths in their rooftop solariums.[3]

The rhythms of day and night and the spectral properties of sunlight are fundamental to our endocrine systems, the timing of our biological clocks, immunologic responsiveness, sexual development, regulation of stress and fatigue, control of infections, and the functioning of our nervous systems.[4] Researcher Richard J. Wurtman, M.D., calls light "the most important environmental input, after food, in controlling bodily function."[5]

Our bodies evolved through millenia of daily contact with sunlight. We need the full spectrum of solar radiation—the infrared (heat), the visible, and the ultraviolet wavelengths—in order to thrive. Different wavelengths stimulate different aspects of our physiology, all playing a vital role in our functioning.[6] Furthermore, our reactions to light are seldom confined to one organ, but demonstrate the interconnected nature of the human body. Inhabitants of extreme northern latitudes, where the winters are long and dark, have identified a "sunlight starvation syndrome." It is characterized by weakened muscles, chronic irritability, frequent minor illnesses, and fatigue.[7]

Though light was once thought to affect us only via our eyes, it is now known to act through our skin and even to reach the brain directly through the skull. Its influence is not limited to the sighted; experiments with blind persons showed that they were able to perceive the presence of light even when there was no accompanying heat or ultraviolet radiation.

Ultraviolet (UV) light is a biologically crucial component of sunlight, but we rarely receive it indoors. It is virtually absent from incandescent lighting, shielded in standard fluorescent tubes, and virtually blocked by normal window glass and eyeglasses. UV radiation has been found to stimulate blood circulation, lower blood pressure, prevent rickets, increase protein metabolism, lessen fa-

[3]Linda Clark, *The Ancient Art of Color Therapy* (New York: Pocket Books, 1975), p. 28.

[4]Hastings, *Health for the Whole Person*, p. 286.

[5]Richard J. Wurtman, "Biological Considerations in Lighting Environments," *Progressive Architecture*, September, 1973, pp. 79-81.

[6]Hastings, p. 286.

[7]Lynne Lohmeier, "Let the Sun Shine In," *East West*, March, 1987, p. 41.

tigue, stimulate the glands, stimulate white blood cells, increase the release of endorphins, and make possible the production of vitamin D, thus increasing absorption of calcium and phosphorous.[8] Moderation is advised, however; overexposure to UV can cause sunburn, skin cancer, cataracts, and dry, wrinkled skin.

Prudent daily exposure to sunlight, unfiltered by windows or eyeglasses, is the most direct solution to UV underexposure, even for dwellers of polluted cities. When this is not practical, UV radiation can be brought indoors via windows made of UV-admitting plastic or via fluorescent lights that include a UV component. When Dr. Alfred V. Zamm built a "healthy house" for himself, he used regular window glass in most of the house, but created an enclosed sun porch with plastic windows. "The plastic was set in removable aluminum frames so that in the summer the area could be screened, and in winter enclosed by plastic, allowing the porch to be flooded with sunlight rich in ultraviolet all year round."[9]

Sunlight contains what we perceive as a balanced distribution of the visible wavelengths of light. Indoor lighting, however, tends to be unbalanced; incandescent lights favor the orange/red end of

THE LIGHT SPECTRUM

the spectrum, and ordinary "cool-white" fluorescent tubes emphasize the yellow/green portion. A few manufacturers, however, produce a fluorescent tube that delivers a range of wavelengths approximating the color balance of sunlight. Several experiments have compared the effects on people of these full-spectrum fluorescent lights with those of cool-white fluorescent lights. In different experiments, full-spectrum fluorescent lighting was found

---

[8]Birren, p. 35
[9]Alfred V. Zamm, M.D., *Why Your House May Endanger Your Health* (New York: Simon and Schuster, 1980), p. 158.

to increase calcium absorption, lessen visual and central nervous system fatigue, improve visual acuity, and decrease hyperactivity. (See Resources, p. 56, for full-spectrum light sources.)

But even the best imitation of sunlight is not the real thing. Researcher John Ott recommends six hours a day of exposure to natural daylight. It needn't all be direct sunlight, and you needn't be outdoors to get it. Natural living consultant Debra Lynn Dadd suggests,

> You may sit on a screened porch, under a shade tree, or even indoors next to an open window. Try to set up a work space with natural light, on a porch or patio, or make a point of eating meals out of doors, or taking breaks for walks during the day.[10]

The daily and seasonal shifts of sunlight affect us, too. For example, early morning and late evening sunlight is red-orange

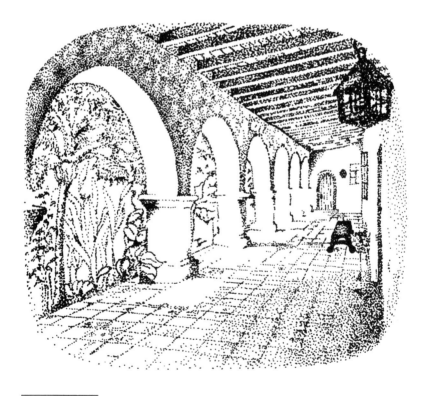

---

[10]Debra Lynn Dadd, "Book Review: *Light, Radiation, and You,*" *Everything Natural,* September/October, 1985, p. 9.

and low in intensity, while noon sun is bluish and high-intensity. Consequently, those combinations of color and intensity appear comfortable to us. Departures from them—bright, warm lighting or dim, cool lighting—appear unnatural and make us feel ill at ease.

As winter approaches, we respond to the shortening of days. Some people show signs of going into hibernation: sleeping more, becoming sedentary, craving carbohydrates, putting on fat, and avoiding social interaction. In many cases, this state is accompanied by feelings of lifelessness, depression, and despair. This condition, now called Seasonal Affective Disorder (SAD), appears to stem from the combined effects of shortened periods of daylight and lack of exposure to full-spectrum light. Regular outdoor walks often reverse the sense of debilitation. Where this is inconvenient or insufficient, SAD patients are being treated by daily exposure to banks of full-spectrum lights, with dramatic positive results.

Light also acts on our well-being as a source of information about the world. We become disoriented if we cannot see outdoor light and thereby lose touch with the time of day, changes in the weather, or a sense of direction. Lighting that is too bright can misinform us, making our surroundings look flat. Abnormal lighting conditions, such as light coming from below us, may make us uneasy. Unnaturally colored light sources cause vague feelings of discomfort; under bluish-white light, people believe they are ill because they look unwell.

The uniform levels of lighting that are common in modern offices are usually unnecessary. Our organisms are not well adapted to monotonous conditions, and accommodating to them produces fatigue.

> People require varying, cycling stimuli to remain sensitive and alert to their environments. Comfort and agreeableness are normally identified with moderate, if not radical change, and this change concerns brightness as well as all other elements in the environment. If overstimulation may cause distress, so may severe monotony. . . . The road to monotony leads to visual efficiency but to emotional rejection; while the road to contrast, though it may lead to emotional acceptance, may impair good visual performance; thus, the place to meet is at the crossroads![11]

---

[11]Birren, p. 24.

Natural lighting is the most effective way to achieve these variations. In addition to going outdoors, we can benefit by bringing daylight indoors via windows, skylights, solariums, atriums, and courtyards.

Under artificial light, variation in the visual field can be created by providing "ambient light" of comfortable but lesser intensity, and "task lighting" at spots that require higher lighting levels. The contrast between ambient and task lighting should not be so great as to cause eyestrain, and glare and annoying distraction should be avoided. Variety in available light sources and the ability to control them is also important.

By varying lighting from one area to another, we can combat monotony and enhance the desired mood and function of each location. In an office, bright lighting is appropriate at desks, but we need a break from that intensity when we are in hallways or the employee lounge. At home, kitchen lighting should allow us to read a cookbook or to slice vegetables, not fingers, but dining room lighting can be low and warm, enhancing social interaction and the appearance of food.

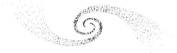

How does sunlight enter your environment? Are you aware of the sun's movement across the sky when you are at home or at work? Which rooms does the sun first shine into in the mornings? Where does sun shine at midday? Which rooms receive evening light? Do those patterns suit your lifestyle and preferences? If not, what changes could you make?

Fantasize your ideal relationship to the sun. Do you feel energized by being awakened by the rising sun? Does watching the sunset from the bathtub give you an incomparable feeling of relaxation? Would you enjoy eating meals outdoors with friends in good weather? Do you want to work in a room with indirect sunlight? Let your mind roam freely, recalling places you've loved, your favorite experiences of sensuality, concentration, relaxation, and so on, and the luminous settings for those feelings.

Notice also your responses to light through skylights, in sunspaces, through glass doors, and through windows of various

kinds. Be aware of the different qualities of direct sunlight, dif-
fused light, and reflected light.

Now look at your indoor lighting. What are the light sources,
and who controls them? Are your rooms washed uniformly by
overhead light fixtures? Does the lighting type, level, and color
reflect different activities in different areas? What is your favorite
kind of light for reading, eating, conversation, working?

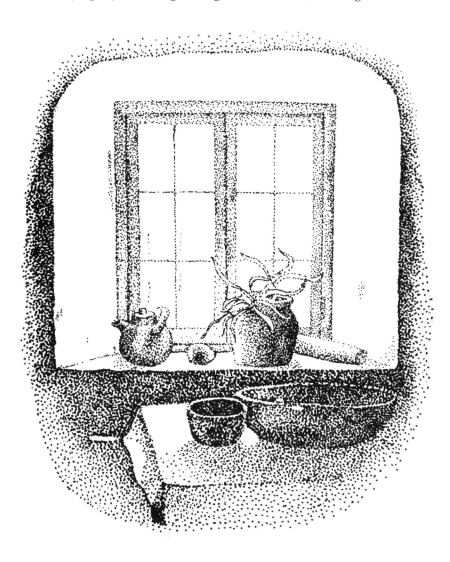

Exploring lighting can open new realms for you. Light needn't always shine directly on the subject; sometimes light reflected off a wall or ceiling makes more peaceful, subtle background illumination. Light shining through a translucent shade can create a special focus. Light softened by a diffusing grid can fall gently on faces around the dinner table. And candlelight can deepen the relaxation and sensuousness of bathing.

Cristina Ismael experimented with the lighting for a tai ch'i class she taught. She was bothered by the cold, sterile fluorescent-lit classroom she was in, so she turned off the overhead lights and used an incandescent lamp and numerous candles. These changes "produced sufficient light and gave the whole atmosphere a softer, gentler, note—very much in keeping with the meditative feeling of tai ch'i. . . . As people walked out of [harshly-lit] rooms into this 'tai ch'i environment' they became quieter and more relaxed. Softer lighting seemed to make people less self-conscious and more receptive. This change also produced a greater amount of interaction among the students, and they began helping one another, rather than comparing themselves to each other."[12]

RESOURCES

Environmental Systems, Inc., 204 Pitney Rd., Lancaster, PA 17601; (717) 394-3182. (*Ott-Lite*; a full-spectrum, radiation-shielded fixture with UV).

Duro-Lite Lamps, Inc., 9 Law Dr., Fairfield, NJ 07004, (800) 526-7193, ext. 5316. (for a list of dealers near you that sell Vita-Lite full-spectrum fluorescent tubes).

Bob Corey Assoc., P.O. Box 73, Merrick, NY 11566; (516) 485-5544. (mail order house for Vita-Lite full-spectrum fluorescent tubes).

The Ion and Light Co., 2263 ½ Sacramento St., San Francisco, CA 94115; (415) 346-6205. (Duro-Lite tubes, full-spectrum Neodymium bulbs, and air purification equipment; consultation on light, color, and ozone technology).

Healthful Hardware, P.O. Box 3217, Prescott, AZ 86302; (602) 445-8225. (Chromalux full-spectrum incandescent bulbs; see also listing in Chap. 11 Resources).

---

[12] Ismael, *The Healing Environment*, p. 73.

· CHAPTER · 8 ·

Color

*Color has the ability to serve man's physiological and psychological
needs and to keep him on an even keel in times of stress.*

—FABER BIRREN

Color is one of the most powerful elements in our environment;
it is typically the first thing we notice when we enter a room.
Color can alter the apparent size and warmth of a room, evoke
memories and associations, encourage introversion or extroversion, induce anger or peacefulness, and influence our physiological
functioning. Changing a room's colors may provide the best health
payback for invested time and money; it's easier to change colors
than to change a room from north-facing to south-facing.

By becoming aware of our responses to color, we can orches-
trate the spectrum of colors around us to enhance our well-being
and harmonize with the desired use of each area. Margaret Walch,
Director of the Color Association of the United States, says, "I
think most people are color-deprived. People have real color
needs, just as they have food needs."[1]

From the perspective of evolution, our color sense is a per-
ceptual aid that has allowed us to adapt to our environment. Col-
or adds dimension to a world that, visually, would otherwise
consist only of light and dark, form and motion. With color we
can better tell the time of day, the ripeness of fruit, the identities
of various plants and animals, and our state of health. Individual
colors and their relationships in groupings tell us more than we
are consciously aware of; they can impart a sense of order where

---

[1]Leslie Kane, "The Power of Color," *Health*, July, 1982, pp. 36-39.

otherwise chaos might reign; they can produce harmony, indicate the season, or evoke spiritual states.

As early as Neanderthal times, color was apparently used for its sacred powers and to invoke aid and protection. Primitive African priests painted traditional designs on cave walls in colors selected for their symbolic healing value.[2] Ancient Greeks and Egyptians used colors in healing.[3] And in the Middle Ages, colored cloth was used to treat disease.[4]

In Europe, stained glass church windows with sunlight streaming through in reds, purples, greens, blues, and yellows were credited with many cures.[5] The special quality of colored light could fill a congregation with a sense of mystery and exaltation. Leonardo da Vinci said, "The power of meditation can be ten times greater under violet light falling through the stained glass window of a quiet church."[6]

Color reaches us deeply and immediately on many levels. Researcher Kurt Goldstein hypothesizes that "a specific color stimulation is accompanied by a specific response pattern of the entire organism."[7] Color affects muscular

---

[2]Betty Wood, *The Healing Power of Color* (New York: Destiny Books, 1984), p. 11.

[3]Clark, *The Ancient Art of Color Therapy*, p. 66.

[4]*Ibid.*, p. 91.

[5]*Ibid.*

[6]Alex Jones, *Seven Mansions of Color* (Marina del Rey: DeVorss & Company, 1982), p. 117.

[7]Birren, *Light, Color, and Environment*, p. 19.

tension, brain wave activity, heart rate, respiration, and other functions of the autonomic nervous system. It arouses emotional and esthetic reactions and associations, both pleasant and unpleasant. And it can bring us to a transcendent state of calm and elevation.

Color was once thought to reach us and act on us only through our eyes. Recent research indicates that we may have a "radiation sense" independent of conscious vision that acts by way of our eyes and skin. Several experiments have shown that colors produce physiological effects on the blind just as they do on the sighted. Sighted subjects wearing blindfolds also show different responses to different colors.

Although there are individual differences in color preference and association, and cultural differences in color symbolism, colors have fairly uniform effects on people within the Western European tradition.[8] Red and blue are the two color "poles," in terms of human response. Red increases blood pressure, respiration rate, heartbeat, muscle activity, eyeblinks, and brain waves, while blue lowers all of these measures. Green or yellow-green produces a neutral response.[9]

Similarly, experimenters have grouped colors into "centrifugal" and "centripetal" ranges.[10] Centrifugal colors are the ones we think of as warm—yellow, peach, pink, orange, and red. They cause us to direct our attention outward, and are conducive to muscular effort, action, and cheeriness. Centripetal colors are the blues, greens, greys, and turquoise. They foster an inward orientation and are appropriate for sedentary activities and those that rely on the eyes or the brain.

Opinions differ as to how to match these qualities with different temperaments. Many color healers and interior designers advise using the color environment to balance the personality, suggesting blues and greens, for example, to calm active or anxious people. But some color psychologists recommend just the opposite. "Excitable people are not necessarily better off with subdued colors, as they can make them feel bottled up; likewise quieter folk can feel very irritated in brash, trendy surroundings. . . .

---

[8]Kane, p. 36.
[9]Birren, p. 19.
[10]*Ibid.*, p. 31.

[O]ften to put a sad, depressed person in too-bright surroundings only makes them retreat even further into their shell."[11] "In small children, a pacific environment and pacific attitude may serve only to increase tension and produce irritability. Here bright color may relieve nervousness by creating an outward stimulus to balance an inner and wholly natural fervor."[12] In other words, an extrovert may be content in a bright, colorful environment, while an introvert may be most at peace in a sedate setting.

On the other hand, you may wish to color your environment to balance out other aspects of your life, giving you a psychic boost. If you live surrounded by sandy desert, you might favor intense colors. If your job requires a lot of activity and extroversion, your home can help you relax and recharge with blues and greens. If you work in an office in a gray building on a gray street, some orange and red highlights at your desk might perk you up.

When choosing colors for a given room, look first at the amount of daylight that enters that room and the warmth or coolness of that light. A dim, cool room can be noticeably warmed by highlights of reds, oranges, or yellows, and vice versa. Consider, also, the use of the room; in each room, the main color should be appropriate to the room's function. Blues, causing introversion, tend to suppress conversation and would not be recommended for social areas. Peach stimulates the appetite and might be appropriate for eating areas. Red, as a tension producer, would be a poor choice for a negotiating room.

In each area, we need some contrasts of dark and light, dull and bright. We need variety as we move from one room to another. We need balance between warm and cool, active and passive. At the same time, we need harmony, unity, and order. Color researcher Alex Jones recommends a maximum of three colors in a room, with highlights of a single, bright color; variety can be produced by changing intensity, value, and texture.[13]

Use your instincts. The colors you like best will probably do you the most good. Putting up with colors you don't like can sap your energy, no matter how healing someone says they are. With

---

[11]Wood, p. 50.
[12]Birren, p. 31.
[13]Jones, p. 98.

the most intense colors, apply moderation; any color can be overdone.

Our eyes are most comfortably adjusted by neutral, non-distracting, cool colors. Too much white causes glare and constricts the pupil. Bright colors and high contrast can result in eye fatigue. These factors are important in areas where people perform visual tasks. When people look up from their work, soothing colors and pleasing views help to relax the eyes.

Generally, we seem most satisfied when color combinations reflect those found in nature. According to Nader Ardalan, nature produces both analogous color harmonies and contrasting color harmonies. Analogous colors are those found adjacent to each other on the color wheel. "Autumn colors scale red through orange, yellow, gold, brown, and purple. The leaves of trees scale yellow-green, green, blue-green. . . . [A] yellow nasturtium will scale toward orange in the center to yellow-green at the stem."[14] Analogous colors reinforce color emotions by supporting and enhancing one another.

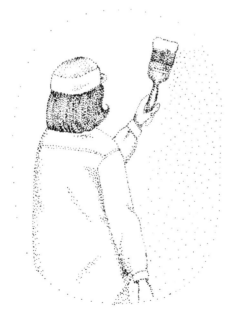

[14]Nader Ardalan, *The Sense of Unity* (Chicago: The University of Chicago Press, 1973), p. 50-51.

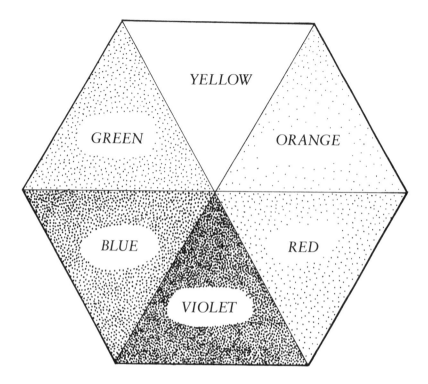

Contrasting colors are opposites on the color wheel; they heighten each other's intensity. In nature, we often find violet flowers with yellow centers and blue birds with yellow-orange highlights in their wings. A brilliant orange sunset grades into the deep blue sky. Use of contrasting colors allows us to balance the warm and the cool, the active and the passive.

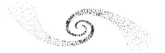

The best way to discover your relationship with each color is to experience and explore it directly. Since color is a phenomenon of the mind, you can do that without leaving your chair. Relax, close your eyes, and breathe easily. Start with pure red: see it all around you, feel it within you, breathe it in and out. Notice how it feels, how it affects your body, mind, emotions, and spirit. Where do you feel it most strongly? You may find images, sounds, sensations, and memories coming up. You may even feel like making sounds or movements. Follow through with these urges; they are

all aspects of what red means to you. When you feel finished with red, breathe deeply, let it go, and let a pure white light wash through you, cleansing and rebalancing you.

One at a time, do the same exercise with the other colors of the rainbow—orange, yellow, green, blue, indigo, and violet—always imagining them in their purest form. You might also try white, black, silver, gold, and various tints and shades such as pink, peach, turquoise, mauve, and burgundy. Each color can be an intense experience; don't feel obliged to try them all at one sitting.

Respect the insights you have about each color. Your own reactions tell you which colors are pleasant, stimulating, healing, suffocating, and so on. Accepted versions of their symbolic or healing properties may help you to understand your reactions, but don't give them precedence over your inner knowledge. You have a unique set of memories, needs, and sensitivities, and your greatest good comes from heeding them.

With that caveat, I will summarize some basic beliefs about color healing (much of which is anecdotal, not experimentally verified), symbolism, and psychology. In general, red, orange, and yellow are considered the "yang" colors; they are stimulating, vitalizing, warming, and dilating. Blue, indigo, and violet are the "yin" colors; they are restricting, cooling, contracting, and astringent. Green is neutral—the balance point in the spectrum.

Red

Red induces excitation, stimulation, and warmth. The color of blood and fire, it is often associated with primitive states and emotions (anger, passion). It is the color of willpower, strength, and vitality. Though it has some associations with disaster and martyrdom, in most cultures it is seen as a positive, creative, life-giving color.

Red stimulates and invigorates the physical body. It increases circulation, muscular activity, blood pressure, respiration, nervous tension, heart rate, and hormonal and sexual activity. It stimulates the nervous system, liver, adrenals, and the senses in general.

Red encourages outer-direction, aggression, and excitation, and overcomes inertia, depression, fear, and melancholy. It counteracts "spaceyness," bringing one into the present and planting one's feet firmly on the earth.

Red is not recommended for anxious people, the emotionally disturbed, or the easily irritated.

In the environment, the stimulation of red can be helpful where physical exercise is the focus or where people lack initiative. It is best used as a highlight color, and should be used with care because of its reactive and impulsive effects. Red should be avoided where calm and rest are desired—in bedrooms, study areas, and meditation rooms. Its irritating quality also makes it a poor choice for eating areas, as people will tend to eat in a hurry and not digest their food well.

Yellow

Yellow vitalizes and accelerates mental activity and feelings of joy. It is the color of the sun, and symbolizes enlightenment, divine power, immortality, happiness, intellectual power, and mental creativity.

Yellow raises blood pressure, pulse, and respiration, though not as strongly as does red. It stimulates the muscles and nerves, and is often helpful for the skin.

Yellow can relieve depression, tension, and fear, and soothe mental and nervous exhaustion. It is generally seen as a cheerful color, but it can be overexciting to an active, irritable condition.

As a mental, creative color, yellow is good to use in libraries, study areas, or any place where mental pursuits will be undertaken. Blue or violet used in conjunction with yellow will help to balance its overstimulating effect.

Blue

Blue, the color of sky and water, symbolizes inspiration, creativity, spirituality, truth, revelation, wisdom, serenity, loyalty, and faith. It is associated with harmony and the highest plane of love.

Blue lowers blood pressure, pulse rate, heartbeat, muscle activity, eyeblinks, and brain waves. The effect is restful and sedating, bestowing quietude, gentleness, contentment, and composure.

Blue counteracts impulsiveness, violence, and restlessness. It soothes mental agitation and cures insomnia. It can induce withdrawal, causing one to center in the inner world.

Blue in the environment has been found to reduce hyperactivity in schoolchildren significantly, but it would be a poor choice for a social area since it may suppress conversation. A blue room is actually experienced as cooler than a warm-colored or neutrally-colored room at the same temperature. The bedroom is a good place for blue's calming, relaxing effect. And its spiritual qualities make blue (along with indigo and violet) a good choice for meditation and contemplation areas.

Orange

Orange is the combination of yellow (wisdom) and red (physicality, action, and power), and therefore is seen as more disciplined and practical than red. It symbolizes optimism, courage, enthusiasm, and confidence.

Orange normalizes the body and replenishes depleted vitality. It is a powerful physical tonic and mental stimulus, promoting energy and exuberance. A social color, it is well used in community centers, meeting places, family rooms, or rooms used for entertaining guests.

As the color of ideas, orange is also good to use in areas for creative study. It is an appetite stimulant, and can be used where this effect is desired. As a universal healer, it can be used in hospital rooms and intensive care units. Touches of orange in the environment can counteract depression and humorlessness.

Too much orange can be overbearing and lead to a tendency to overindulge. Nervous people should avoid orange. Orange is best used in moderation, as a highlight color.

Green

Green is a mixture of blue (spirituality and calm) and yellow (wisdom). It is associated with nature and its cycles of birth, death, and transformation. It symbolizes both abundance and unripeness, and represents balance, harmony, growth, healing, love, peace, and hope.

Sometimes called "the master healer," green affects the whole system and is especially beneficial to the central nervous system. It has a sedative effect, relieving irritation and exhaustion. Green subdues nervousness and tension and is good for concentration and meditation. It soothes emotional disorders and nervous headaches.

Green can be irritating, however, if it is dominant and monochromatic; nature is abundant in greens, but they vary greatly in hue. Green can also be overwhelming for people who need stimulation or who are not in balance.

Calming green is best used in areas that are for rest and relaxation. It is ideal for bedrooms and hospital rooms. Its qualities of peace and harmony also make it a good choice for rooms where political matters are dealt with.

Purple

Purple combines red (physicality, action, and power) with blue (spirituality and calm). It suggests dignity and is therefore often used for rituals, spiritual or political. It both accelerates and sublimates all the processes of the body, mind, and spirit. Purple induces relaxation and sleep, lowers body temperature, and decreases sensitivity to pain. It is also a stimulant, however, increasing the activity of the veins.

Indigo

Indigo symbolizes intuition, devotion, and spirituality. Though it can be cool and dispassionate, "a true indigo, like the evening sky, suggests inner light of a quality to offset cooler attributes."[15] It is uplifting and has a hint of mystery.

Indigo can be helpful in the environment if one tends to be overly practical or intellectual. If one is too spacey, however, indigo would be inappropriate. Indigo's spiritual and protective qualities make it a good color for a meditation area. But it is powerful and should be used sparingly.

---

[15]Wood, p. 98.

Violet

Violet symbolizes humility, creative imagination, and spiritual realization. It is seen as equivalent to the highest and most evolved state of consciousness.

Violet has been used to soothe serious mental conditions, overexcitement, and overstimulation, restoring peace and calm to the high strung. It also induces a deep, relaxed sleep.

Violet's development of the imagination makes it a good choice for areas where creative projects are undertaken. Its spiritual aspect recommends it for meditation and contemplation rooms. Richard Wagner placed violet curtains in front of himself when he wanted to compose spiritual music.[16]

White

White carries all the qualities of all the colors. It is associated with both life and death, and stands for wholeness, purity, and innocence. White added to any color is said to give it greater spiritual qualities. White visually intensifies other colors when placed beside them. White stands for positivity and banishes negativity. It has connotations of coolness, purity, and cleanliness.

Black

Black is associated with the primordial darkness, negativity, and death. It can have an ominous presence. However, it also suggests strength, absorbs and restores energy, and restricts and protects. Black can be a good color for introspection, but it is hard to live with constantly or in quantity.

Pink

Pink is a tint of red. It works on the mind, evokes loving feelings, and is regarded as a universal healing color. It has a restful, tranquilizing effect but is not recommended for use around psychotics or temperamental people, as it may further disturb them.

---

[16]Jones, p. 117.

Turquoise

As a combination of blue and green, turquoise exerts a tranquilizing, cooling, relaxing effect and is an aid to nutrition and repair. Turquoise decreases brain activity and is therefore helpful to the mentally overactive.

Magenta

Magenta is a combination of red and violet. It is a general body stimulant and an emotional stabilizer.

Scarlet

Scarlet is red with a touch of blue. It is a general body healer and brain stimulant, and counteracts discouragement.

Brown

Brown symbolizes earth, and as such is the color of balance for light-headed people. It aids concentration and acquisition of knowledge but should be used discriminatingly, as it can have a heavy effect.

Gray

Gray represents persistence and spiritual struggle, death and rebirth. A depressed person should not use it as a major color in the environment.

Gold

Gold is the color of the sun and is rich and warming.

Silver

The color of the moon, silver is cool and delicate; it represents peace. As an accent, it can be an aid to creativity.

CHAPTER 9

The Thermal Environment

The thermal environment ... has the potential for ... sensuality, cultural roles, and symbolism that need not be designed out of existence in the name of a thermally neutral world.
—LISA HESCHONG

Heat and cold are among the most pervasive features of an environment. They strongly influence how we feel in a place, both physically and emotionally. But we tend to take notice of thermal properties only if they are particularly pleasant or unpleasant. A cool breeze on a warm summer day or a fire in the fireplace when we come in from the cold are universally gratifying sensations, while an unventilated, stuffy room can sour any occasion. In this era of thermostatically controlled central heating and air-conditioning, many of us don't think about the range of thermal possibilities and how they may affect our lives and our well-being.

Before we achieved the technological feat of optimum uniform temperature at all points in a building at all times, the meaning of "indoors," the uses of rooms, and people's daily activities took a different form than they do in this country today. In earlier times (and in many non-industrialized areas today), people adapted their lifestyle to the thermal conditions of the hour or the season, often migrating within and around their buildings to take advantage of the different microclimates. In times of cold, they gathered around a central fire; in heat, they gravitated to courtyards and gardens. In hot climates, people were most active in the cool mornings, and took siestas in the afternoons. Primitive builders used forms and materials that responded appropriately to their climatic conditions: clay and stone in the desert; bamboo and reeds in the tropics.

Only with the advent of the furnace, and later the air conditioner, did people begin to think of buildings as enclosures of comfortably warm or cool air. Subsequent research and technology were aimed at providing thermal environments that demanded as little as possible of people, both physiologically and in terms of involvement with the mechanics. The buildings enclosing those thermal environments were no longer required to temper the climate and ceased to reflect their locale with its daily and seasonal variations.

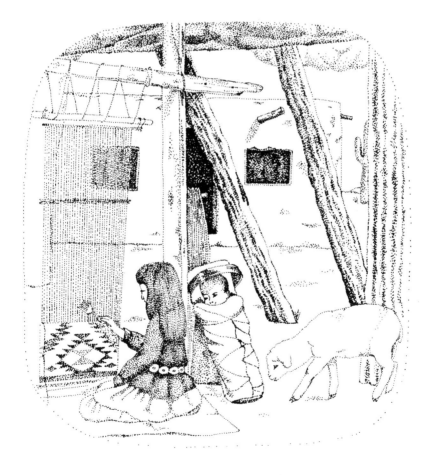

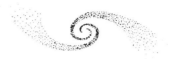

What is your favorite climate? What climate(s) did your ancestors live in? What climate(s) did you grow up in? If you had to choose one or the other, would you rather be slightly warm or slightly cool?

Recall some of your favorite places. What are their climates? In what seasons have you visited these places? Remember the thermal sensations connected to your experiences there.

What is the source of warmth or coolness in each of the places where you spend your time? Who controls it? Does it satisfy you, irritate you, increase your sense of social connection?

Thermally speaking, we humans are composed of a core, which maintains a nearly constant temperature, and a shell, which alters its temperature and heat flow in response to ambient conditions in order to keep the core temperature stable. Our bodies react to extreme cold by increasing heat production, and to extreme heat by secreting sweat. We accommodate moderate temperature variations by changing our bloodflow and the insulating values of our surface tissues.

Our thermal comfort is a product not only of air temperature, but also of the temperatures of nearby surfaces, air motion, humidity, and stratification. There is no one perfect combination of all these factors for several reasons. First, the factors work together; a high temperature can be uncomfortable if the humidity is high and the air is still, yet the same air temperature can be comfortable at reduced humidity or increased air speed. Second, each person has a different comfort standard, depending on age, sex, build, health, ethnic background, hydration, type of clothing, and level of activity. Third, standards vary for an individual from season to season, and differ among people living in different climates. And finally, we may actually need thermal variations in order to function at our best.

HEALTH AND THE THERMAL ENVIRONMENT

Thermal conditions affect our health in several ways. Extremes of heat or cold can be hazardous and even fatal to the elderly, the very young, and others with impaired ability to regulate their internal temperatures.

Cold weather increases the incidence of heart attacks, epileptic seizures, asthma attacks, arthritis flare-ups, headaches, and colds.[1] People who chronically suffer from such ailments are often advised simply to move to a warmer climate. A winter vacation is a less drastic solution, but the shock of returning can often reverse the beneficial effects of having left.

On the positive side, cold can be a vitalizing force to people in good health. Cold increases our metabolism and makes us feel energetic.

Excessive heat, on the other hand, induces sluggishness, impairs mental efficiency, slows reaction time, and hampers our ability to deal with stress. Even if you spend most of your time in air-conditioned comfort, the shock of walking out of a chilled building into the hot outdoors takes its toll. The reverse effect—a sudden chill upon walking indoors—can be just as bad, increasing your susceptibility to illness. The effect can be lessened by keeping indoor temperatures closer to those outdoors (78-80° F instead of 70° F), or by using natural cooling techniques, such as shading, air motion, evaporation, and massive building materials.

Studies have indicated that there is a range of climatic conditions within which human physical strength and mental activity are at their best. Outside this range, efficiency drops, and stress and susceptibility to disease are said to increase.[2] The implied goal is to create environments that do not place any stress on the body's heat-compensation mechanism.

The comfort zone for the average person falls between 69°F and 80°F, and 30% to 60% relative humidity when the air is still. But even within these ranges, stress will result if the air is either motionless or drafty, the temperatures of nearby surfaces cause

---

[1] Norman and Madelyn Carlisle, *Where to Live for Your Health* (New York: Harcourt Brace Jovanovich, 1980), pp. 28-30.

[2] Victor Olgyay, *Design With Climate* (Princeton: Princeton University Press, 1963), p. 14.

uncomfortable body heat loss or gain, one side of the body is significantly warmer or cooler than the other, or the floor-to-ceiling temperature difference is greater than a few degrees.

Lisa Heschong, in her book *Thermal Delight in Architecture,* contends that this goal of creating thermally stress-free environments has been carried too far:

> There is an underlying assumption that the best thermal environment never needs to be noticed and that once an objectively "comfortable" thermal environment has been provided, all of our thermal needs will have been met.[3]

She contends that "neutralizing" the thermal environment cuts us off from enjoying its potential sensuality, cultural meaning, and symbolism. Our ability to use our "thermal sense" to explore the world around us, in all its variability, becomes a part of our sense of vitality. Our health and happiness, says Heschong, depend less on uniformity than on variation in stimuli.

Imagine again the world in which our bodies evolved (see Chapter 3). We were made to be "tuned up" by all the changes around us, perceiving, processing, and responding to myriad useful sensory inputs. Heschong adds, "Our nervous system is much more attuned to noticing change in the environment than to noticing steady states. . . . [U]niformity is extremely unnatural and therefore requires a great deal of effort, and energy, to maintain." By contrast, she describes the "extra delight in the delicious comfort of a balmy spring day as I walk beneath a row of trees and sense the alternating warmth and coolness of sun and shade."[4]

The return to designing buildings in response to climate, and employing "passive" or "natural" methods of heating and cooling, may be as healthy for us as it is for our planet. It not only conserves fossil fuel and reduces pollution but also reintegrates us with climatic cycles, both physiologically and mentally. Our bodies and spirits are enlivened by the shifting conditions, and our daily activities fall into a rhythm more attuned with other forms of life. Naturally heated and cooled buildings typically involve their inhabitants in operating vents, blinds, or shutters, un-

---

[3]Lisa Heschong, *Thermal Delight in Architecture* (Cambridge: The M.I.T. Press, 1979), p. 16.
[4]*Ibid.,* p. 19.

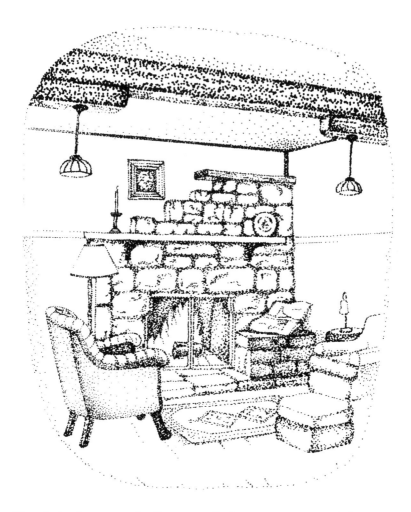

like their thermostatically controlled counterparts. While sometimes resistant at first, people often find that operating such "switches" tunes up their awareness and enhances their sense of integration, of belonging in the larger world of natural phenomena. When we modify natural thermal extremes for our pleasure and health without completely damping out the daily and seasonal changes, we allow our bodies to receive the clues on which they thrive.

Builder Karen Terry describes life in her passive solar heated adobe home in New Mexico: "Living in a solar house is a whole new awareness, another dimension. I have the comfort of a house with the serenity of being outdoors—protected, yet tuned in."[5] Like many people in pre-industrial cultures, Terry migrates within her home, which steps down the hillside: she works in her studio on the cool lower level, eats in the middle level, and bathes and sleeps in the warmest upper level. She says she has a feeling of being connected to natural rhythms.

Janius Eddy, another solar-heated home dweller, adds, "It has made us profoundly grateful that the sun is up there, the center of our universe, warming us up and keeping us alive. That atavistic sense of the elements that early man knew and felt has become part of our lives."[6]

Central heating and cooling have also helped us to forget many of the symbolic tools that people have used in other places and times to increase their sense of comfort. Qualities that suggest warmth include soft fuzzy surfaces, warm earthy colors, mellow aromas, and golden light. Coolness is evoked by running water, wind chimes, cool colors, things that sway in the breeze, lacey latticework, and shade. These suggestive climate-modifiers help us not only to feel warmer or cooler; they also add to the richness of our experience, helping us to notice a breeze or feel cozier around a fireplace. All of our senses are brought into play to heighten our experience of thermal pleasure and wholeness.

Our sources of warmth or coolness, when not hidden as most furnaces and air conditioners are, can also have symbolic meanings that bond us with our heritage and with other people. The hearth is a prime example; it is the traditional center of family life, and it symbolizes warmth, security, and companionship. There is a unique revery induced by gazing at flames or embers. The fire is traditionally the place where the family or community gathers to warm themselves, cook meals, tell stories, and reinforce their ties to one another. Emotional and physical warmth intermingle, and the meaning of the hearth becomes deepened, inspiring affection for the whole place and ritual. The Finnish sauna, the Japanese bath, and the Chinese k'ang (a raised clay platform heated from below) all serve this dual function of providing physical warmth and social contact. This adds another dimension to

---

[5]*Ibid.*, p. 57.
[6]*Ibid.*

the healing properties of the place, since love and a sense of be-longing are among the most important factors in a person's health.

ASPECTS OF THERMAL COMFORT

The right thermal conditions and the right way of achieving them are an individual matter. You will need to evaluate your genetic makeup, physical health, climate, tastes, and lifestyle to arrive at the best fit for you. In many instances, a creative combination of "passive" and "mechanical" tools will meet the widest range of needs. Let's take a closer look at some of the aspects of the thermal environment, and at some ways of modifying them.

Humidity

Relative humidity (RH) indicates the amount of water in a volume of air, compared to the amount which that volume could hold. As air temperature rises, the air can hold more water. Consequently, 50% RH at 100°F is moister than 50% RH at 50°F.

Humidity affects health in several ways. When combined with summer heat, it inhibits sweating, making it harder for us to cool off. We become sluggish and irritable. Hospital admissions and deaths rise during both humid heat spells and wet cold waves.

In cold climates, the winter RH outdoors is often low. When the air is heated indoors, its RH decreases even further. Without added moisture, this dry air (if less than 20-30% RH) can dry out the protective linings of the nose, throat, and lungs, apparently causing increased susceptibility to colds and flu. Studies performed in Europe showed that when indoor RH was increased by 8 to 10%, bringing it to 22 to 50% RH, absenteeism was reduced by 10% for adults and 50% for kindergarten children.[7]

Winter humidity has two additional advantages: humid air feels warmer at lower temperatures than dry air, reducing fuel consumption, and humid air reduces the static charge in the air

---

[7]P. O. Fanger, *Indoor Climate* (Copenhagen: Danish Building Research Institute, 1979). p. 208.

(the sparks that shock you when you touch a metal object after walking across a carpet).

But there is an upper limit to healthy humidity. Excessive indoor humidity is believed to promote the spread of viral infections by providing microorganisms with the warm moisture they need for survival. Humidity above 70% RH is conducive to mold growth; inhaled mold spores can cause endless misery to the allergic and may eventually weaken the defenses of the not-yet-allergic.

If you want to test for RH, you can do so fairly easily with a sling psychrometer, also known as a dry-bulb/wet-bulb hygrometer. They are sold at heating and plumbing supply stores, scientific supply houses, and meteorology stores.

You can influence indoor humidity by altering your habits. Cooking, operating a clothes dryer, sweating, showering, and growing houseplants all add moisture to the air. If your indoor air is too moist, you may wish to isolate and vent such sources of humidity; if it is too dry, you might emphasize them. If these activities are not effective enough, you may wish to alter the humidity mechanically. Many types of humidifiers and dehumidifiers are available. Try to buy a system with a filter that you can clean yourself with a stiff brush and water to combat mold growth in the filter. The manufacturer-recommended practice of adding chlorine bleach or other toxic substances to inhibit mold can cause its own problems by distributing those poisons throughout the air you breathe.

Air Cooling

Many doctors and biometeorologists feel that air conditioning handicaps us by not allowing us to adapt to heat. Dr. Jan. A. Stolwijk, a Yale Professor of Epidemiology and Public Health, says, "I feel it is far better to move the air around than to cool it off. In my opinion, there is nothing so good as the southern ceiling fans, the kind you see in old New Orleans. A gentle air motion downward can be a big help."[8]

There are many ways to cool and ventilate spaces without

---

[8]Julius Fast, *Weather Language* (New York: Wyden Books, 1979), p. 93.

noisy, fuel-consuming chillers. Trees and shrubs can provide shade while adding visual delight. Buildings can be designed or remodeled to reduce direct solar radiation and promote ventilation by such means as overhangs, blinds, and well-placed operable windows. Light-colored exterior walls can be used to reflect heat away from a building. Interior masonry or earth walls will soak up heat from the indoor air. And we can adopt techniques used by traditional builders in hot-arid climates, such as screens, courtyards, and open towers that capture passing breezes and conduct them to the lower floors of the house.

Natural cooling, however, is not always the answer. For hay fever sufferers, a properly filtered air conditioner may be the only solution when pollen counts are high. And many people living in polluted areas need a break from the outdoor air. For such individuals, Sidney J. Heiman suggests the following qualities for "an ecologic air conditioning system":[9]

1. Low air velocity, to avoid draftiness and minimize stirring up of dust and other particulates.

2. A constant flow of air at a median temperature—more tolerable to hypersensitive people than shorter bursts of extreme temperatures.

3. A range of filters to remove gaseous contaminants and microscopic particulates without producing ozone.

4. Isolated motors and fans, installed outside the air-cooling box.

5. Drainage of collected moisture to avoid mold growth.

6. No outside air intake; if outside air is necessary, it should be filtered at the point of intake.

7. Outdoor compressor location, in case of refrigerant leakage.

---

[9]Guy O. Pfeiffer, *The Household Environment and Chronic Illness* (Springfield: Charles C. Thomas, Publishers, 1980), p. 159.

Heating

The equipment that provides heat—and even the type of heat supplied—plays an important role in indoor health. Heating equipment is a major source of indoor air pollution: most gas- or oil-fired furnaces give off fumes and by-products that can cause headaches, dizziness, fatigue, respiratory problems, heart palpitations, and impaired vision, hearing, and brain function; wood-stoves can give off toxic by-products that irritate the eyes, nose, and respiratory system; steam heat can release chlorine into the air; airborne particulates that pass through a furnace or come to rest on an electric resistance heater become "fried dust," releasing toxic gases into the air; and mechanically circulated air stirs up dust and other particles, constantly delivering them to our nostrils.

Every writer on indoor ecology has a favorite heating system, and they're all different. They agree on some basics, though: kerosene space heaters and all unvented gas heaters are deadly and should be eliminated; environmentally sensitive people who have gas- or oil-fired furnaces may need to modify or remove them; and gas- or oil-fired furnaces in new construction should have air intake and exhaust to the outdoors.

If you want to keep your gas- or oil-fired furnace, you can reduce its negative impact with a few measures. Have someone from the utility company test the lines and the firebox for leaks; the tests should involve instrumentation, as odor tests are inadequate. Have a professional adjust the furnace at least once a year. And be sure that you have adequate outside air for combustion in the furnace.

If you are sensitive to the combustion products of gas or oil, and these measures do not significantly lessen your reactions, you might be wise to shut off the furnace and have the gas line capped outside the house. Your other option is to install a new furnace that has intake and exhaust to the outdoors only. If you are in a multi-unit building with a central furnace, you can still get some relief by closing off the vents to your space securely, using a metal foil barrier and foil tape.

When selecting a mode of heating, your first choice might be whether to provide ambient heating or radiant heating. Ambient heating is the norm in most buildings today; it involves heating all the air in the building so that the air can, in turn, heat us. Radiant heating warms people and objects directly without heating the intervening air.

If you elect centralized ambient heating, Alfred V. Zamm, M.D., recommends the heat pump. Heat pumps extract heat from outdoor air, water, or soil and distribute it indoors in winter; in summer the cycle is reversed. Their lower operating temperatures lessen the likelihood of fried dust. They run on electricity, eliminating the problems of gas and oil, and are relatively energy efficient in mild climates (though decreasingly so in colder climates). An outdoor location for the heat pump will avoid the possibility of coolant escaping into the house and will lessen the indoor impact of pump noise (a significant problem).

Woodstoves combine radiant and ambient heating characteristics and can be selected to avoid indoor air contamination. The best stoves are as airtight as possible and have an outside combustion air source to ensure a good draft up the flue. Debra Lynn Dadd advises: "Make sure wood stoves and fireplaces are installed and fitted properly. Fix cracks or leaks in the stovepipe, and keep the chimney and stovepipe clean and unblocked. . . . . Fragrant softwoods such as pine and cedar may give off odors that can be troublesome for some people. Use dry, well-seasoned wood only, because it will smoke less. Do not use the pressed-sawdust logs or paper-wrapped easy-to-light logs sold in grocery stores; they may have been treated with toxic chemicals."[10] In an area where the chimney smoke will contribute significantly to outdoor pollution, it's best to use a different heating method for the sake of everyone's health.

Another heating system that gets good reviews is the hydronic baseboard heater. Hot-liquid electric baseboard heaters release no airborne pollutants or fried dust, due to lower operating temperature. They do not contribute to noise pollution. They provide a steady heat with no drafts, allowing natural air motion to distribute the heat, as compared with using a fan.

---

[10]Debra Lynn Dadd, *Nontoxic and Natural* (Los Angeles: Jeremy P. Tarcher, Inc., 1984), p. 30.

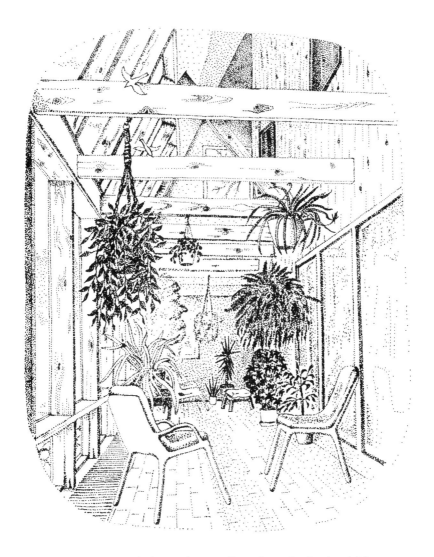

Many experts believe that radiant heat is the healthiest way to warm ourselves. If we look at our evolution again, this makes some sense: the sun and fire both provide radiant heat. Radiant heat travels as infrared rays and "heats differentially, according to the capacity of a material to absorb infrared."[11] It heats people

---

[11]Edward T. Hall, "Let's Heat People Instead of Houses," *Human Nature*, January, 1979, p. 45.

and objects instead of air, and is felt as a gentle, satisfying warmth. Radiant heat is believed to act not only on our surface, where ambient heat acts, but to penetrate to our core as well, activating enzymatic processes in the cells and influencing the central nervous system, the internal organs, and gas exchange. When heated radiantly, we are comfortable at lower air temperatures, increasing muscle tone and inducing a feeling of freshness and vigor. And radiant heat eliminates the need to move masses of warmed air around, thereby keeping our mucous membranes moist and healthy and cutting down on circulated dust. However, since radiant heating systems don't introduce outdoor air or circulate indoor air, humidity and stale odors can build up unless air exchange is provided.

Passive solar heating offers the cleanest and most energy-efficient form of radiant heat. It produces no fumes, consumes no fossil fuels, and reconnects us with natural cycles. There are two important cautions, however, concerning the thermal storage mass: if rock beds or similar materials are used, they may become growing ground for mold, and any stone, masonry, or concrete should be carefully screened for radon emissions (see Chapter 11).

Radiant-floor heating is also healthful and can be used in conjunction with passive solar heating. The advent of polybutylene tubing has caused a resurgence in the popularity of radiant-floor heating. Older systems made with metal piping were notorious for leaks, necessitating costly repairs and often driving up indoor humidity uncomfortably. Polybutylene tubing can be installed in a concrete slab or in a 1½-inch lightweight concrete topping over a wood floor (again, check concrete for radon). The system is quiet, clean, and comfortable, and doesn't blow dust or pollen around. The water that circulates in the tubes can be heated by the sun, wood, electricity, oil, or gas, though fossil fuels may be inappropriate for health reasons. The initial flexibility of this system allows you to indulge your preferences; by spacing tubes closer together in the bathroom, for example, you can be warmer in a place where you tend to be unclothed. The main health caution with radiant floor systems is to avoid floor coverings such as vinyl, carpet, or wood; the heat from the slab can volatilize the cements and the flooring materials, releasing toxic substances into the air.[12] Mortar-set tile, stone, or concrete are preferred (see pp. 122-4).

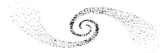

Fantasize freely about your thermal environment, drawing on past experiences as well as preferences that have never been indulged. What would make you feel really good? A warm floor where your bare feet first touch it in the morning? Direct sunlight on your skin in the bathroom? An inglenook for snuggling up with others around the hearth? In summer, where would a cooling breeze help most? Would a garden with a fountain and windchimes be more satisfying than an air conditioner?

Don't limit your imagination by what you think you can do. Once you begin to explore the possibilities, you will find that there are many scales on which you can satisfy your wishes. You are dead only when you lack wishes!

---

[12]Zamm, *Why Your House May Endanger Your Health*, p. 163.

· CHAPTER · 10 ·

Sound and Noise

It is time man realizes that his home can be designed
to acoustic criteria, resulting in a pleasant environment for him
and medically conducive to a state of well-being ...

—LEE E. FARR

As far as we know, human hearing evolved in a relatively quiet setting. Although extremes of heat and cold, dark and light, wet and dry were a normal part of primitive life, very loud noises were the exception. The sounds that were heard all carried meaning to the hearer, and the ability to detect subtle sounds was important for both survival and pleasure. The snapping of a twig, the call of an animal, the tone of the wind, and myriad other sounds gave a constant sonic picture of the state of things. Even relative silence had a gentle, reassuring texture, as occasional subtle sounds reinforced a sense of peace. On the rare occasions when sound crossed the threshold of discomfort—a thunderclap, an avalanche, a volcanic eruption—it carried a crucial message; the "startle" response that was evoked and its concomitant adrenaline rush were entirely appropriate for self-preservation.

Even as civilization advanced, the sonic environment remained fairly unpolluted until recently.

Our colonial ancestor would have heard few sounds, none of them physiologically stressful: conversation of neighbors or sound of churchbells; song of a bird or sigh of wind in the trees; call of the ploughman or blows of the blacksmith at his anvil. Many sounds might have been threatening by reason of the information they contained—rattlesnake whirring, panther crying, Indian warwhoop or rattle of musketry—but none of them was in itself dangerous to health.[1]

Ironically, the situation has now been reversed: in our homes, towns, and cities we seldom escape noise, the sound level is often physically harmful, and the background noise rarely contains useful information. Noise is defined as unwanted or harmful sound. We human beings are engineered to "read" sound, but not to endure it. While our sense of hearing can provide a rich connection to the world around us, it has become for many people a source of constant insult—mental, physical, and emotional. We deal with unwelcome sounds by tuning them out, but evidence now suggests that the damage to our health continues nevertheless.

Loss of hearing is one of the most direct results of noise. Though gradual hearing loss with age has been assumed to be natural, we now know that industrialized civilization has caused significant acceleration of hearing loss. Dr. Samuel Rosen, between 1961 and 1963, compared the hearing of American city dwellers to that of the remote Mabaans of Africa. While the city

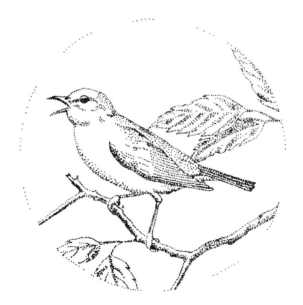

---

[1]James Marston Fitch, *American Building* (New York: Schocken Books, 1972), p. 132.

noise level averaged 60 to 75 decibels (db),[2] the sound level in the Mabaan villages was usually below 40db. Rosen's team found the Mabaans' hearing to be remarkably superior to the Americans'; the difference became marked in the age group of 30 to 39 years, and among the 70 to 79-year-olds 53% of the Mabaans could hear sounds audible to only 2% of New Yorkers.[3] Another study comparing Londoners to West Africans found that West Africans in their seventies had hearing superior to Londoners in their twenties.[4]

In addition to hearing loss, a complex and growing list of ills is being blamed on noise. The body responds to noise with high blood pressure, headaches, tension, hyperactivity, poor digestion, ulcers, fatigue, cardiovascular disease, decreased immunity, neurological disorders, and disturbed sleep. Irritability, lack of concentration, moodiness, poor work performance, and mental disturbance can also result. High general noise levels interfere with conversation, reading, listening to music, or contemplation—all activities that would otherwise contribute to our well-being. Sudden noises, though they convey no immediate danger, are registered by our bodies as warning signals; our blood pressure and heart rate soar, our breathing speeds up, our muscles tense, and hormones are released into our blood. When exposed to repeated loud noises, the body is put into a perpetual state of "startle response," with muscles chronically tensed; this can lead to overall fatigue, diminished reflex reactions, and accident proneness. Over time, one's ability to respond to real danger can become impaired.

In existing diseases, noise can worsen the condition in real and immediate ways. "Any disease which may be associated with an emotional charge requires as part of the therapy a calm, relaxed, quiet environment."[5]

Psychologically, the impact of sound is not entirely a function of its loudness. A noise is more easily tolerated if it is under one's

---

[2]A decibel is a measurement of the intensity of sound. The decibel scale is logarithmic; an 80db sound is ten times greater than a 70db sound. An increase of 3db amounts to a physical doubling of the sound level, but it is barely perceptible.

[3]*Ibid.*, p. 156.

[4]California Department of Consumer Affairs, *Clean Your Room!* (Sacramento: California Department of Consumer Affairs, 1982), p. III.P.10.

[5]Lee E. Farr, "Medical Consequences of Environmental Home Noises," in *People and Buildings,* ed. by Robert Gutman (New York: Basic Books, Inc., 1972), p. 209.

control, if it has some relation to the listener, or if it is perceived as contributing to a positive result. Thus, your own lawnmower is less annoying than your neighbor's, your baby's cry is more meaningful than a random noise, and fan noise seems tolerable when the fan is cooling the room. The annoyance potential of sound is increased by reverberation, intermittency, inappropriateness, or unexpectedness. Annoyance is also cumulative; day-long noise exposure makes one more likely to be irritated by a single loud noise in the quiet evening.

As ambient noise levels have increased over the last several decades, city dwellers have paid the greatest price. In cities, we are exposed to traffic noise, street repairs, construction, subways, sirens, loud music, and airplanes. But suburb and country noise have increased as well—farm equipment, highway noise, chain saws, lawn mowers, airplanes, sonic booms, gunfire, and snowmobiles all contribute to noise pollution.

In city or country, the indoor sounds of most modern homes provide little escape from noise. Dishwashers, vacuum cleaners, refrigerators, televisions, fluorescent lights, electric shavers, food processors, ventilating fans, garbage disposals, electric mixers, and knife sharpeners all produce disquieting noises that create general nervous tension, resulting in health damage and interpersonal strain.[6] In the normal kitchen, useful mechanical devices can drive the sound level into a dangerous range. "A tired, taut person will certainly not leave a kitchen pleasantly relaxed; nor do the roars, squeaks, whirrs, and whines issuing from it lead to contemplation of pleasant meals by those who are waiting."[7] Even the quieter indoor noises can be irritating. The intermittent droning of the refrigerator, the humming of fluorescent lights, and the background whine of television can create a numbing, dulling effect. Sound researcher Steven Halpern says that if you shut off a background noise source, such as a fluorescent light or a refrigerator, "...you can feel a difference in the pressure in your chest. What most people notice is that they will be much more energized when some of these devices are off."[8]

---

[6]Steven Halpern, *Sound Health* (San Francisco: Harper & Row, 1985), p. 16.

[7]Farr, p. 208.

[8]Debra Lynn Dadd, "Sound Health: An Interview With Steven Halpern on Sound and Wellness," *Everything Natural*, July/August, 1986, p. 3.

Workplaces have their own cacophony. In the office, buzzing lights, ringing phones, conversation, office machines, computers, and the decreasing use of real walls between work areas all make concentration difficult. In factories, the loud, incessant noise of machines can cause hearing damage and mental fatigue.

The human ear can detect sounds over a range from 0db to 150db. Normal human conversation falls between 50db and 75db. Extensive exposure to levels in excess of 85db usually causes permanent hearing loss. The following table indicates the average decibel levels for a range of common noises; actual values may very widely.

SOUND LEVELS[9]

Sound Source	Decibel Level
moderate rainfall	50
"quiet" apartment	50-60
chirping birds	60
bathroom ventilating fan	63
washing machine	65
television (at 8 feet)	68
dishwasher	69
vacuum cleaner	70-75
stove vent fan	70-85
garbage disposal	72-78
busy traffic	75-85
window air conditioner	80
electric shaver	85
jack hammer	100
chain saw	100
motorcycle	100
amplified live rock music	90-130
air raid siren	130
jet engine at take-off	120-140

[9]compiled from: Halpern, p. 14, and Farr, p. 204.

In the wilderness, the average sound level is 15 to 20db. In a farm area, the level rises to 30 to 35db. Suburbs and small towns generally experience 35 to 45db. And ambient city noise ranges from 45 to 75db. Environmental Protection Agency (EPA) data indicate that between 1950 and 1970 the number of noise sources in the United States grew much more rapidly than did the population.

Steven Halpern, in his book *Sound Health,* aptly illustrates the rise in urban noise levels: before World War I, the brass bell on a fire truck was enough to clear traffic from its path; in the 1930s, the bell was insufficient to rise above ambient noise, and the siren was introduced; by 1964, siren volume had to reach 88db at 50 feet to be heard; today's urban noise level requires that sirens reach 122db—louder than jet engines or firecrackers. At this level, physical pain and permanent ear damage are likely.

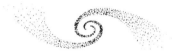

For a few moments, close your eyes and notice the sounds around you. What sounds come to you from outdoors, and which from indoors? Which are pleasant, and which are unpleasant? How many are under your control? Notice the constant background noise as well as the intermittent sounds. Which sounds give you messages, and what do they tell you? Watch your physical and emotional reactions to each sound—tension, relaxation, annoyance, reassurance, numbness. Notice the total sound level—the aggregate volume of all the sounds around you: is it generally peaceful, buzzing, roaring? Does the sound level rise and fall? How many of the sounds you hear are caused by people, by other animals, by the elements (wind, rain)?

What are your favorite sounds? Is there something you don't hear that you wish you could hear? Something you'd feel better without? If you want to take this further, cast back to some of your favorite memories and places. Are there sounds associated with these memories—a creaking gate, splashing water, a screen door banging, a crackling fire, driving rain, a grandmother's humming?

Your sonic environment will change over the course of the

day and will differ from place to place. Your reactions may also change with time of day, degree of stress, and other factors. Try this awareness exercise in different places at different times, and see what you begin to learn about your needs and preferences.

HEALING YOUR SONIC ENVIRONMENT

Though many noise sources are out of our control, we can improve our immediate sonic environments once we are aware of them. Sound control tactics fall into several categories. Their priority depends on your immediate problems, wishes, and resources. The most straightforward way to avoid noise that is beyond your control is to get away from its source. Barring that, there are landscaping and building construction techniques that will reduce the level of noise reaching you indoors. You can also cut back your use of indoor noisemakers and sonically isolate or dampen those you find necessary. Unavoidable noises can be quieted by your choice of interior finishes. And, finally, you can introduce pleasant sounds, either to mask unwanted ones or to increase your pleasure and relaxation.

Avoidance. If you are considering a move to a new home or job, take the ambient noise level into account. In the case of airports, freeways, and other major noise polluters, avoidance is the best policy for your health and sanity. Several studies have found that deaths, admissions to mental hospitals, drinking problems, high blood pressure, learning disabilities, heart disease, and many other ills are much higher among people living near airports than among those in quieter neighborhoods—often two to three times higher.

Don't stop at avoiding the worst offenders. Map out the whole area you are considering, locating major industries, highways, railroads, mass transit, flight paths, hospitals and fire stations (sources of regular siren noise), major intersections, bus stops, school yards, parking lots, playgrounds, construction sites, logging operations, shopping centers, fairgrounds, air bases, power substations, transformers, major transmission lines, and so on. If you have a particular location in mind, visit it at different times of day and on different days of the week to witness the sound levels. In addition to avoiding noise, you can seek out pleasant sounds. Consider which locations are likely to provide the sounds you prefer—birds in the trees, wind, a stream, ocean waves, human voices.

Landscaping. Noise is nearly impossible to avoid altogether, and often other constraints cause us to be in less-than-perfect sonic surroundings. There are still many ways to improve a given situation. If you have some land between your building and a noise source, you can lessen the intensity of noise reaching the building. Earth berms (planted mounds of dirt) and rows of thick trees or shrubs will reflect and absorb sound. A fence of concrete or masonry will do the same. If you are planning a new structure, placing it partially below ground level will also help—either by building into the ground or by cutting back the earth and placing the building in a "crater." Any of these techniques can be used alone or in combination.

"Acoustical" plantings serve many needs at once: they are pleasant to look at and be around; they help clean and cool the air; they hide the noise source from view, lessening its psychological impact; and they can attract birds which add a pleasant sound of their own. The best shrubs for absorbing noise are those with many thick, fleshy leaves and thin leaf stalks that allow flexibility and vibration. When planting tree belts, the taller the trees and the wider the belt, the more effective they will be. It takes a small forest to eliminate unwanted sounds, but lesser plantings can lower noise levels. Such planting screens should be as close as possible to the noise source (the street, for example) to absorb the sound and deflect it away from your building. Deciduous trees work better in summer, but are less effective in winter, than evergreens.

Construction. The best barrier to sound transmission is a massive partition; concrete or masonry will absorb more airborne sound than lighter construction. Where such materials are inappropriate, the next best technique is to provide "structural discontinuity" in the wall. This can be done by staggering the studs in new construction, by adding a second wall or "skin" to an existing building and leaving an airspace between the two walls, or by hanging the

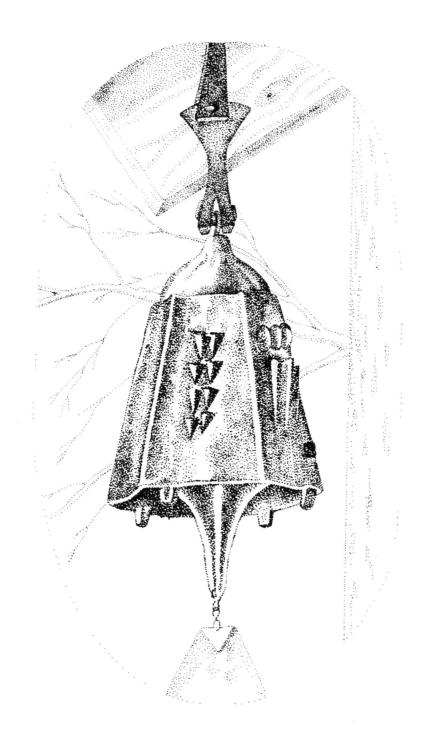

interior wall finish with resilient metal channels made for this purpose. Such methods work by minimizing the travel of vibrations through the structural members to the inside.

Another way to reduce entering sound is to seal up the building for greater thermal efficiency. The same insulation, double-pane windows, weatherstripping, and caulking that lessen heat transfer will also dampen noise from outdoors. Sealing cracks is more important than it may appear; you might have concrete walls and insulating glass, but all it takes is a small, unprotected slit around a door or between structural panels to allow noise to invade your structure.

Indoor Noise Control. Evaluate the noise sources in your home and workplace in terms of their loudness, annoyance, and usefulness. There may be some items you could do without altogether, replacing a food processor with a knife, an adding machine with an electronic calculator, a garbage disposal with a compost pile, an electric shaver with a razor, or an air conditioner with natural cooling and ventilation. You may decide to honor your sanity simply by not using ten noisy machines at the same time.

You can reduce noise levels considerably by putting padding under typewriters, blenders, and similar machines. Larger equipment—refrigerators, furnaces, washing machines—can also be installed on special vibration mounting. The infamous buzz of fluorescent lights can be lessened by installing higher quality ballasts or remote ballasts, and by relamping when the tubes begin to hum. When you buy new appliances or equipment, compare brands and models for sound output; don't be fooled by the old myth that the noisier a machine is the better a job it does.

You can also design a room so as to isolate the noisemakers. Some items can be placed in insulated cabinets. At home, a sound-isolated utility porch is a great place to put the washer and dryer, freezer, furnace, and even the refrigerator. In an office, the photocopier, postage meter, blueprint machine, and coffee maker can all be in a separate room with a door. Noise-generating areas can be distant or insulated from areas where quiet is crucial to relaxation or performance.

People who live or work together need to become more aware of each others' sonic spheres. Education about noise pollution can form the basis for friendly communication about ways to reduce everyone's stress level. People can make trade-offs or reach compromises about their noise production that will remove many sources of physical and interpersonal tension.

Absorption. Once a noise has been generated inside or has entered from outside your building, you can lessen its intensity by using absorbing materials. Soft, porous materials like carpets, upholstery, drapes, heavy textile wall hangings, and acoustic panels and tiles will reduce or dampen interior noise levels. Where noise is a problem, minimize hard, nonporous surfaces such as plaster, glass, concrete, and sheet plastics that reflect sound.

Healing Sounds. Too much success in limiting indoor sound could become a different kind of problem. Extreme, sustained silence is as unnatural to us as constant noise. Deprivation of any of our senses results in mental and physical strain. Although we desire a peaceful environment in which we can relax or concentrate, total silence is usually not the goal.

As with other aspects of our surroundings, the greatest satisfaction comes not just from eliminating noise problems, but from introducing or enhancing the sounds that soothe, delight, or encourage us, and that help us to feel our wholeness. Once you become aware of the kinds of sounds you prefer, you can find a variety of ways to provide them. Any pleasant sound can also act as "masking noise," diminishing your awareness of less desirable noises.

One approach is to increase the amount of desirable sound immediately outside your home or workplace. In most places, you can at least put a bird feeder at the window to attract some delightful little creatures who might chirp for you. With more room, you can install a bird bath, and hear not only warbles but splashes as well. And if you really like birds and have the freedom to landscape, plant trees and shrubs that attract birds. Any shrub with berries will provide food for songbirds, particularly dogwoods, hawthorns, mahonias, mountain ash, pyracanthas, toyon, and most viburnums. Many species of trees will feed and shelter songbirds: birch, oak, ash, maple, white pine, beech, cedar, white spruce, hemlock, flowering dogwood, cherry, palmetto, winterberry, sycamore, willow, alder, and crab apple. Squirrels and chipmunks may also be attracted by these trees.

Other trees can be planted for the sounds they themselves make when the wind blows through them. Bamboo and casurina require only slight breezes to create rustling or whistling sounds, respectively. Quaking aspen, oak, poplar, and pine all make gentle sounds in the wind, and their leaves or needles crunch nicely when walked on.

Breezes can create a variety of sounds, depending on what you hang in their path. Wind bells, wind chimes, flags, pinwheels,

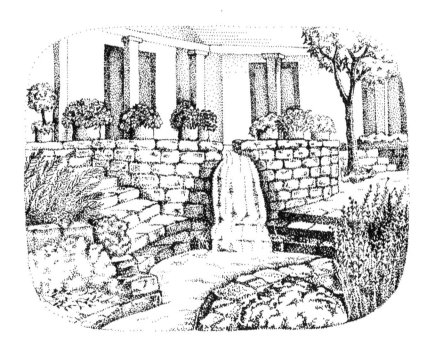

paper streamers, wind flutes, or anything else you dream up can keep you in touch with the movement of air outside.

Water, too, provides myriad opportunities. A pond can be home to croaking or peeping frogs and other life forms. A bubbling fountain or a splashing waterfall makes soothing sounds. Fountains and waterfalls can be simple or lavish, depending on your budget, but they are not only for the rich.

If you lack the outdoor space for such amenities, many of

these sounds can be brought indoors. You can keep crickets or frogs as pets in pleasant terrariums. You can hang a wind chime inside an open window. You can even install an indoor recirculating fountain or waterfall. An array of restful recorded nature sounds is also available; in your own home or workplace, you can tune in to birds, crickets, frogs, whales, ocean waves, rainstorms, streams, and other sonic environments.

Music is a powerful tool that is increasingly used in healing. It has the potential to relax us and to reach beyond our analytical minds directly into our emotional centers. The organized, purposeful aspect of music can serve as an antidote to the disorganized auditory pollution we tolerate. Carefully created and selected music can aid relaxation, concentration, creativity, meditation, muscle response, digestion, mood, healing, and positive mental states.[10]

Not all music is healing, however. Several studies have found that rock music can be physically and mentally damaging. The loud volume of rock music is blamed for significant hearing losses in teenagers and young adults. Even at harmless volumes, the standard rhythms of rock music have been found to confuse the body and weaken the muscles.[11] Classical music is generally less harmful than rock, but it is not always healing either. The best way to select healing music is to become aware of your subtle physical and emotional responses as you listen to a piece. Simply liking a piece of music may not be the best indicator of its healing potential; you might find it to be emotionally rousing but physically tension-producing. Notice your breathing; shallow, random breathing suggests disharmony, whereas deep, regular breathing implies that you and the music are in resonance. Notice also your degree of muscular tension before and during listening. If the music induces overall tension or tightening in certain areas, chances are that it's not the piece you need to refresh you. Become more aware of subtle changes in heart rate, mental activity, eyeblinks, emotional response, and so on. As you learn to recognize your reactions to sounds, you will be better able to create a positive, health-promoting sonic environment. You can even ask your body

[10]Halpern, p. 9.
[11]*Ibid.*, p. 70.

what kind of music or sounds it would like, to help attune and heal it.

Don't overlook the enormous value of making your own healing sounds. Whether you sing in the shower, hum over your work, play folk songs with friends, or weave soulful melodies on your flute, the immediacy of the vibrations and your creative involvement bring an added dimension to music's healing properties.

· CHAPTER · 11 ·

Indoor Air Quality

*The average home today contains more chemicals
than were found in a typical chemistry lab
at the turn of the century.*
—DEBRA LYNN DADD

Not long ago, when people talked about making their buildings "safe," they were usually referring to security against dangers from outside like burglary or earthquakes. Now, growing numbers of people are concerned about hazards generated from within their homes and workplaces—airborne gases and particles that undermine their mental and physical health. Recent cases of indoor air pollution in new office buildings and schools have been widely publicized; upon moving into a shiny new building, occupants complain of nausea, headaches, lethargy, puffy eyes, stuffy noses, coughing fits, and a long list of other ailments. The phenomenon, known as "Sick Building Syndrome," is usually attributed to two factors: increased use of volatile synthetic materials, and decreased ventilation rates aimed at energy conservation.

Although the natural atmosphere has always carried bacteria, molds, viruses, pollens, spores, and dusts, nothing in our makeup prepares us for some of the toxic substances we now encounter daily. The nature and volume of these poisons is so new that we don't know what's hit us. Some air pollutants are two to one hundred times more concentrated indoors than outdoors. While some contaminants are detectable by smell upon first exposure, many are odorless and colorless, and thus go unnoticed. Even those with characteristic odors are often ignored; after the initial exposure, our olfactory sensors lose their sensitivity to a given smell. In many ways, the sleuthing out of indoor irritants is a whole new game.

Many who have been negatively affected by "sick" buildings apparently recover their health after improving the quality of the air they breathe. But increasingly, people who become chronically sensitized to minute concentrations of toxics develop escalating allergies known as Environmental Illness or Multiple Chemical Sensitivity (EI/MCS). EI/MCS has caused heated debate in the healthcare community, with some practitioners maintaining that it is either a nonexistent or a psychologically based problem, while others try to help patients with debilitating symptoms and unclear etiologies. Highly sensitive people can have problems for years that appear to be viral or psychological in nature before suspecting that they may be reacting to something in their environment.

Dr. James A. O'Shea, former president of the American Academy of Environmental Medicine, says that roughly four to five million Americans suffer from chemically induced environmental sensitivities, but that only about five percent have been treated for it. "Many people are walking around with environmental illness and don't even know it yet."[1] William J. Rea, M.D., estimates that environmental illness already affects "a good twenty percent of the population, and the number is going to get higher."[2]

It is easy to think that sensitivity to toxic substances in the environment is the problem of the unfortunate few, and that if we're not incapacitated we have no need to be concerned. However, there is a growing belief that highly sensitive people may be early warning signals to us all.

According to natural living consultant Debra Lynn Dadd,

> Each of us is born with an inherited ability to process substances that enter our bodies, both beneficial and foreign or harmful. Our inherited ability sets a certain built-in limit as to how much exposure to potential toxics we can endure without harm. As long as the amount of toxics coming into our bodies stays under that level and our tolerance threshold is not exceeded, our bodies will adapt and metabolize or excrete the poisons with no ill effects. It is when our bodies become overloaded that

---

[1]Peter Fossel, "Sick-Home Blues," *Harrowsmith*, September/October, 1987, p. 49.
[2]*Ibid.*

symptoms and disease occur. Once that level is reached, even the slightest exposure can produce symptoms.[3]

Dr. Alfred V. Zamm, a physician who treats people with environmental sensitivities, divides the population into three categories:

1. People who are sensitive to environmental pollutants, are aware of the problem, and are taking action to improve their situation;

2. People who may have environmental sensitivities and don't realize it, but who are "depressed much of the time, tired without good reason, weak and logy and slow-thinking";

3. People who appear to be unaffected but who are probably not reaching their potential because they are surrounded by "incipient poisons."[4]

That leaves none of us untouched. Furthermore, people in the "unaffected" category often move suddenly and catastrophically into a "sensitive" category when the effects of the toxic environment reach a point the body can no longer tolerate. The annals of environmental illness are filled with stories of previously productive, happy people who have been crippled by a single sensitizing episode or a cumulative dose of a toxic substance. Their lives often become complicated as sensitivity to one chemical spreads to related substances.

Suzanne Randegger, editor of *Environ* magazine, urges:

The more we can avoid the small or unnoticed toxic exposures, the less likely we are to become increasingly sensitized to chemically related substances until we reach the overload stage, where our bodies react indiscriminately.[5]

Since most of us spend 90% of our time indoors, we need to be careful about what we surround ourselves with. The National Academy of Sciences estimates that indoor air pollution already

---

[3]Debra Lynn Dadd, "Basic Toxicology," *Everything Natural*, January/February, 1987, p. 17.
[4]Zamm, *Why Your House May Endanger Your Health*, p. 11.
[5]Suzanne Randegger, "Q & A Dept.," *Environ*, Summer, 1988, p. 23.

adds from 15 billion to 100 billion dollars to our nation's annual medical bills.[6] Furthermore, indoor pollutants have been found to affect productivity, stress levels, sense of well-being, and absenteeism. In the long run, it is cheaper to make our buildings as pollution-free as possible.

Unfortunately, the magnitude of the problem is not matched by the volume of useful research findings. Though recommended maximum exposure levels exist for various pollutants, no one knows what levels, if any, of indoor pollutants are acceptable over the long term. Little is known about the interactions and synergistic effects of multiple contaminants. For many substances, appropriate measurement techniques are still being developed. And we're only beginning to understand the health effects of indoor air pollutants and ways of controlling them. But the problems are great enough that we can't wait until all the data are in from scientific studies underway or not yet begun. We need to act now, relying on our own rationality and instincts, on the research that has been done, and on our direct experiences and those of others.

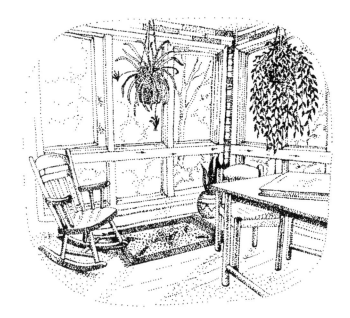

[6]Suzanne and Ed Randegger, "A Real Rocky Mountain High?" *Environ*, Fall/Winter, 1986-87, p. 23.

The point of this chapter is not to produce anxiety or paranoia; such a state might be more of a health hazard than unclean air. The point is to help you get a handle on things; awareness and education can lead to positive action. If you are a silent sufferer, you can learn to alter your environment and lifestyle to greatly relieve your mysterious ailments. If you are relatively unaffected, you can take precautionary steps to better assure your continued health and perhaps even improve your present functioning. The goal is to help you create an environment where you can refresh and recharge yourself, unencumbered by insidious assaults.

INDOOR AIR QUALITY HAZARDS

The following summaries of the major indoor air pollutants will acquaint you with their basic characteristics. If you suspect that any of them pose a problem in your environment, refer to the Resources section at the end of this chapter for sources of more detailed information.

Formaldehyde

Considered by some to be the most worrisome indoor pollutant, formaldehyde gas is toxic to most forms of life. Thad Godish, Director of the Indoor Air Quality Research Laboratory at Indiana's Ball State University, says that formaldehyde perils lurk in the vast majority of American homes.[7] Although people's levels of sensitivity to formaldehyde vary widely, repeated exposure can increase one's sensitivity. Many people—especially mobile home dwellers—have had to abandon their homes because of highly irritating formaldehyde levels.

Possible Health Effects. Results of continued or excessive formaldehyde exposure have included irritation of the mucous membranes of the eyes, nose, and upper respiratory tract; skin irritation and rashes; chronic headaches, lethargy, and memory

---

[7]Suzanne and Ed Randegger, "Formaldehyde and Health," *Environ*, Fall-Winter, 1986-87, p. 6.

lapses; sleep disturbance; irritability, paranoia, depression, disorientation, and moodiness; chest pains and heart problems; cold or flu-like symptoms including coughing, watery eyes, swelling of the throat, and breathing problems; nosebleeds; nausea; menstrual problems; and possible cancer and other chronic or long-term effects.

Perhaps most serious is the sensitizing effect of formaldehyde. Overexposure, whether occurring suddenly or over time, can result in extreme sensitivity to minute concentrations of formaldehyde and, some say, to other substances as well.

Sources. The greatest amounts of indoor formaldehyde come from a few products: medium-density fiberboard or particleboard products (such as subflooring, paneling, solid-core doors, and cabinetry), urea-formaldehyde foam insulation (UFFI), and much contemporary furniture (solid wood as well as upholstered), all of which may contain urea-formaldehyde. Lesser emitters that may increase formaldehyde levels are synthetic carpets, carpet glue, drapes, office partitions, oil-based paints and resins, permanent press fabrics, plastics, ceiling tiles, and combustion (tobacco smoke, gas stoves, woodstoves, and kerosene space heaters).

Urea-formaldehyde resin can outgas[8] for the life of the product, but phenol-formaldehyde resin is more stable and therefore less hazardous. For that reason, some experts consider products containing phenol-formaldehyde resin, such as exterior-grade plywood, to be relatively safe for healthy people.

Remedies. According to Godish, source removal is the only effective way to reduce high concentrations of formaldehyde; all the major sources must be identified and removed. Replace particleboard subflooring with tongue-and-groove boards or exterior grade softwood plywood (except in cases of sensitivity to softwood or to plywood adhesives); choose metal or hardwood cabinets; select solid wood, metal, or old (already outgassed) furniture; replace particleboard or hardwood plywood wall paneling with decorative hardboard, drywall, or plaster.

Alternatively, it is possible to seal in some of the formaldehyde

---

[8]"Outgassing" is the gradual release of gasses from a substance.

fumes. A water-based sealer or nitrocellulose-based varnish can be used effectively on particleboard subflooring, hardwood plywood panelling, particleboard shelving, cabinet joints and edges, countertop undersurfaces, and unfinished furniture. Such sealants may need to be reapplied every few years. A more durable barrier is aluminum foil sealed with foil tape.

If UFFI is outgassing into your home, your best protection is to remove it as completely as possible. After removal, Godish recommends that you treat all cavity wood surfaces with a 3% solution of sodium bisulfite and allow it to dry before installing new insulation. If gypsum wallboard is adjacent to the UFFI, you may need to replace it as well; formaldehyde has been known to seep into wallboard, continuing to contaminate the house. If it is impractical to remove the UFFI, you can caulk or spackle holes and cracks in the insulated walls to reduce passage of formaldehyde. Applying two coats of a vapor-barrier paint or installing canvas-backed mylar or vinyl wallpaper will also help reduce outgassing (see cautions about paint and wallpaper on page 125).

Because heat and moisture accelerate formaldehyde emission, formaldehyde levels can be controlled somewhat by lowering temperature and humidity. Ventilation can also lower formaldehyde levels by dilution. Air filtration may offer additional relief; use specially impregnated charcoals or an activated alumina medium impregnated with potassium permanganate, or both, and replace them as needed.

The level of formaldehyde outgassing from a given source will decrease over time. However, after several years some products still give off enough formaldehyde to cause health problems.

Indoor formaldehyde levels can be determined relatively easily and inexpensively. Some state health departments will perform free tests, or you can purchase a test kit and do the test yourself (see Resources for mail-order companies).

Combustion Products

The products of burning common fuels can include carbon monoxide, carbon dioxide, nitric oxide, nitrogen dioxide, and hydrocarbons. In homes, the worst offender is gas; many researchers agree that a healthy house should not even be connected to a gas line. Alfred V. Zamm, M.D., rates gas second only to cigarette smoke as the worst home pollutant. Zamm observes that many women who spend a lot of time in the kitchen become sensitive to gas; they acquire a depression that psychiatry can't cure, but the depression often disappears when their gas range is replaced with an electric one.[9]

Carbon monoxide (CO), an odorless, colorless gas, is the most widely recognized combustion product pollutant. The National Center for Health Statistics estimates that 2% of the U.S. population (over 4.5 million people) is exposed to indoor CO in excess of the EPA's standard for outdoor air.

Possible Health Effects. For many people, headaches, dizziness, and fatigue can result from eight hours around a normal gas stove. Higher concentrations of CO can cause flu-mimicking symptoms, nausea, convulsions, mental confusion, loss of alertness, impaired heart function, and death.

Nitric oxide (NO) and nitrogen dioxide (NO$_2$) can reduce lung function and increase colds and bronchitis. They have been implicated in long-term respiratory problems, heart disease, and cancer. Hydrocarbons cause cancer in lab animals and can damage the liver, respiratory system, and nerve tissue.

Joseph T. Morgan, M.D., says that gas can have a sensitizing effect similar to that of formaldehyde: ". . . one of the best ways to induce chemical sensitivity is to be subjected to long-term exposure to natural gas in combusted and/or uncombusted form."[10]

Sources. The main indoor sources of combustion products are tobacco smoke, wood- and coal-burning stoves, fireplaces, gas ranges, self-cleaning electric ovens, automobiles idling in attached garages, water heaters, clothes dryers, and furnaces or heaters that burn charcoal, gas, kerosene, oil, or wood. Combustion products enter indoor air at open flames or via rusted flues, defective pipes, or failed welds. Improperly adjusted or vented heating devices pump out large volumes of CO. In this country, about 200 people die each year from poisoning by space heaters, usually kerosene-

---

[9]Zamm, p. 23.
[10]Joseph T. Morgan, M.D., letter to the editor, *East West*, July, 1987.

fueled. But, according to Zamm, even a normal gas oven operating at 350°F for one hour with the vent fan on can cause kitchen air pollution comparable to a heavy Los Angeles smog. Without a fan, CO and NO_2 can zoom to three times those levels or more.[11]

Remedies. The most complete way to eliminate combustion products is to remove all gas-burning appliances and have the gas line capped off at the street. An electric range or a magnetic-induction range can be substituted for a gas range. Homes without gas appliances have significantly lower levels of combustion products than do homes where gas is burned. Debra Lynn Dadd says, "I have seen many clients do everything I recommend except remove the gas from their homes, and their health problems remain. But almost as soon as they turn off the gas appliances, they start feeling better. It's amazing."[12]

Short of removing all gas, you can reduce combustion pollutant levels somewhat. Gas ranges should have hoods vented to the outside, and the fan should be operated any time the range or oven is used. The more powerful the fan and the more enclosing the hood, the better. An open window will also improve air exchange.

When possible, isolate combustion appliances in a room that can be closed or sealed off from the living space. Gas furnaces that are located outside the building—or that use outside combustion air and exhaust it directly to the outdoors—pose minimal health hazards for most people. Maintain your gas appliances for optimum functioning: clean burners and blocked flues, fix cracks and leaks in pipes, and keep appliances adjusted; a poorly adjusted gas stove can give off thirty times more CO than a properly adjusted one.

Woodstove pollution can be minimized indoors by selecting an airtight stove and keeping the flue clean and in good repair. One expert points out that there's no such thing as an airtight flue, and recommends eliminating woodstoves and fireplaces altogether. For most people, however, such an extreme is not necessary.

---

[11]Zamm, p. 23.

[12]Debra Lynn Dadd, *The Nontoxic Home* (Los Angeles: Jeremy P. Tarcher, Inc., 1986), p. 173.

Radon

Radon is as old as the mountains; it is one of the indoor pollutants that we can only partially blame on modern living. It is a colorless, odorless gas that is a byproduct of decaying uranium in rocks and soil. The gas seeps out and decays into radioactive "daughter" products which can then lodge in the lung tissue. Experts disagree about the risks of low to moderate exposures, but it is believed that the combined effect of radon and other indoor pollutants (notably cigarette smoke) may significantly increase hazards. In 1987, the EPA found 20% of the 9,600 homes it surveyed in 10 states to be contaminated with potentially health-threatening levels of radon gas.[13]

Possible Health Effects. The EPA considers radon to be the leading cause of lung cancer in non-smokers.[14] EPA statistics suggest that 10% of all lung cancers in the United States are caused by radon; the Consumer Federation of America attributes up to 30,000 lung cancer occurrences per year to radon.[15] And the lung cancer risk from radon may only be the tip of the iceberg of adverse effects. Spending a week—or even a year—in a building with moderate radon contamination probably wouldn't cause cancer. But 20 years in such a house might well increase your risk.[16] Unfortunately, carcinogens such as radon don't cause noticeable short-term symptoms.

Sources. The radon content of rocks and soils varies greatly. Soils high in radon have been found in parts of Pennsylvania, Washington, New York, New Jersey, Florida, Texas, Maine, and Vermont. Radon concentrations in rocks range from very low in sandstone to fairly high in granite and even higher in alum shale.

In areas where radon is abundant in the soil, it is sucked directly into the lower levels of the house, especially through

---

[13]"EPA Finds Radon a Widespread Health Threat," *Chemical & Engineering News,* August 10, 1987, p. 18.

[14]Lois Ember, "EPA Compiling Data on Extent of Indoor Radon Hazard, "*Chemical & Engineering News,* August 17, 1987, p. 22.

[15]Lynne Lohmeier, Ph.D., "Indoor Pollution Alert," *East West,* March, 1987, p. 45.

[16]LaFavore, Michael, "The Radon Report," *Rodale's New Shelter,* January, 1986, p. 31.

cracks in a basement wall or a concrete slab on grade. It can also enter through sump pumps, drains, and fittings around underground utility pipes. Radon-bearing well water can contribute to indoor radon levels as the water splashes from faucets, showerheads, and washing machines. Decorative rock walls around fireplaces, or used as thermal mass in passive solar heated buildings, may introduce radon to the indoors. Concrete, cinder block, or bricks made with radon-bearing materials can also increase radon levels. In Colorado, radon-rich tailings from uranium processing mills were used in the foundations of several schools and more than 4,800 homes.

Remedies. Control methods fall into four categories: ventilation, filtration, removal or sealing, and prevention at the site-selection and building-design stage. For a test of radon levels in your building, contact your state agency that deals with radon, or your regional EPA office.

Increased ventilation can remove radon gas and lessen its concentration indoors. Increasing the air pressure inside a building will discourage the entry of radon (or any other) gas from outside. Whether natural or forced ventilation is used, be careful not to reduce indoor air pressure, thus pulling more radon inside. But even well-designed ventilation won't solve the problems of high radon concentrations.

Filtration is controversial; some say that an electrostatic precipitator will reduce radon levels by removing radon-bearing dust from the air; others say that filtration is useless since radon is a gas.

If radon-bearing soil is a problem, increasing foundation drainage, ventilating crawlspaces or under slabs, or covering earthen basement floors or crawlspaces with non-radon-bearing concrete can reduce infiltration indoors. Sealant applied to the foundation and to interior masonry will limit the release of radon.

For a new structure, careful site selection, material choice, and ventilation design can assure low radon levels from the outset. In Sweden, a piece of land must be tested for radon before a new house can be built. If high radon levels are found, the builder must follow government guidelines to ensure an uncontaminated house.

Asbestos

Called "one of the most pernicious indoor pollutants,"[17] asbestos problems have been publicized for years. A fine, fibrous material, asbestos is widespread in walls, ceilings, and elsewhere in many modern buildings. Urban autopsies find asbestos in lung tissues in almost every case.[18]

Possible Health Effects. Asbestos can cause malignant tumors in the chest lining or abdominal cavities and increases the risk of cancer of the gastrointestinal tract and the larynx.

Sources. Asbestos has been used inside buildings for fireproofing, decoration, and thermal, electrical, and acoustical insulation. It has been widely used in schools, making school children and school employees especially vulnerable. Asbestos is harmless as long as it stays where it is applied. The hazard arises when fibers are released into the air or water, eventually lodging in the lungs or gastrointestinal tract.

Remedies. In most cases, undamaged asbestos products are best left alone. Some asbestos applications can be sealed to keep fibers from sloughing off into the air. Where asbestos-containing products are crumbling or damaged, repair or removal is recommended; removal must be performed carefully, however, or it can produce even higher levels of asbestos in the air.

House Dust

House dust is composed of molds, bacteria, mites, pollen, human and animal hair and dandruff, textile fragments, leftover food, pesticides, and decomposed material. Forty percent of the allergic population reacts to house dust. Of those, one quarter react to the house dust mite.[19]

---

[17]California Department of Consumer Affairs, p. ES9.
[18]*Ibid.*
[19]Fanger, p. 196.

Possible Health Effects. Since house dust can include particles of almost any allergen, reactions to it cover a full range of allergic responses: runny nose, sneezing, scratchy throat, coughing, fuzzy thinking, and even hives. As a carrier of bacteria and viruses, it can also aid in spreading colds and flu.

Sources. As evidenced by its composition, the sources of house dust are everywhere. Animals, plants, people, fabrics, insects, and anything else that sloughs off fibers or particles can contribute to dust. Though some amount of dust cannot be avoided, it becomes a problem whenever it is stirred up, re-entering the airflow and eventually the lungs. Housecleaning stirs up dust. Neglected furnace filters constantly recharge the air with dust. Sitting on upholstered furniture, moving drapes, and shaking rugs all stir up dust.

Remedies. Ventilation and air filtration will reduce the volume of dust particles in indoor air. Frequent housecleaning is a must, but special care is needed to keep from re-introducing settled dust into the air. Avoid dusters, dry mops, and brooms. Use a damp cloth to clean moldings, sills, light fixtures, shelves, and the tops of door and window jambs. Open the windows when cleaning to blow out any dust you may raise. Vacuum cleaners are tricky; they suck up dust, but the finest particles blow back out through the filter bag. One solution is a central vacuum system that collects the dust outside the living space. Some special vacuum cleaners have highly efficient particle filters.

You can avoid providing places for dust to collect by limiting carpets, drapes, wall hangings, window sills, dust-collecting nooks and ledges, and open-front cabinets.

Mold

Molds exist in the air throughout the year, in varying concentrations. Mold spores are light and easily carried by air currents. Most of us don't realize how many damp, mold-growth-encouraging places there are indoors until we start looking.

Possible Health Effects. In people sensitive to mold, symptoms can include a stuffy, runny nose, sore throat, dry eyes, bronchial troubles, fatigue, headaches, and depression. Exposure to large doses of mold may also sensitize people not previously allergic to it.

Sources. A little moisture and darkness is all that molds need to proliferate. Mold grows in damp basements, bathrooms, closets, mattresses, carpets, and old upholstered furniture. In the kitchen, it thrives between the sink and the wall, around the bottom of the cold water pipe, in chopping boards, on the refrigerator door gasket, and in the surplus water tray at the bottom of self-defrosting refrigerators. In bathrooms, it grows in tile grout, around the sink, on walls, on the back of the toilet tank, and on the shower doors. Old newspapers, books, or magazines can grow mold, as do flower pots, the surfaces of houseplant soil, and any decaying plant material.

Remedies. Get rid of old damp, moldy materials. Clean moldy areas with a borax solution or diluted Zephiran. Ventilate the bathroom and other moisture-producing areas well; hang towels where they can dry. Put a layer of sterile potting soil or crushed stone over houseplant soil surfaces. Install louvered doors on damp closets. If you have a damp basement, air it out and keep it dry. If water gets into the basement via a roof downspout, extend the leader to carry rainwater away and downhill. You may also want to waterproof your basement or install a dehumidifier. If you use a humidifier elsewhere in your home, clean it frequently with water and a stiff vegetable brush. Avoid future mold growth by ventilation, humidity control, sunlight, and regular cleaning of vulnerable areas.

Lead

Lead contamination pervades the modern environment. Typical Americans have 100 to 1,000 times the lead in their bodies that their prehistoric ancestors had. No safe level for lead exposure has been demonstrated.

Possible Health Effects. Chronic exposure to low levels of lead produces permanent neuropsychological defects and behavior disorders.

Sources. Inside buildings, the major source of lead is leaded paint. Since lead is now illegal as a paint component, the hazard mostly exists in older buildings. It is particularly dangerous where paint is cracked or peeling, especially where children inadvertently eat it. Some lead may also enter drinking water via old lead pipes or newer copper pipes with lead-containing solder at the joints.

Remedies. Lead paint can be removed, but special precautions should be taken to avoid breathing its dust, letting the dust spread throughout the building, or leaving residue that could enter food or the air. In new plumbing installations, copper pipe can be joined with lead-free solder or friction fittings.

Softwoods

"Natural" isn't always best, especially for people sensitive to softwood vapors. Softwoods (pine, spruce, cedar, redwood, and other conifers) contain volatile resins that outgas for years. Wood panelling, cedar closets, fireplace wood, and Christmas trees can all produce reactions in sensitive people.

Air Ions

Negative air ions have received a lot of attention as a quick fix for problems ranging from lethargy to arthritis to impotence. But the subject is complex, and scientific research has produced few reliable results to date.

Air ions are atmospheric molecules that have become charged by the loss or gain of an electron. They are constantly being formed and are constantly recombining to neutralize their charges. Air ions are naturally produced by cosmic rays, radioactive soil elements, weather fronts, moving water, and wind. Euphoric feelings around waterfalls or before thunderstorms are attributed to high negative ion concentrations. In open country, under favorable weather conditions, there are typically 1,000 air ions per cubic centimeter of air; in large cities there are approximately 200 ions per cubic centimeter of air.[20]

Researcher Albert P. Krueger, M.D., says that lab experiments support four conclusions:

—Ions are biologically active, affecting living matter from bacteria to human beings.
—Depletion of ions in the air may increase a person's susceptibility to illnesses like respiratory infections.
—An increase in ions and particularly in the ratio of negative to positive ions may be useful in the treatment of burns and respiratory diseases.
—Conditions in urban centers, characterized by air pollution outdoors and artificially controlled climates indoors, lower the total number of small ions in the air and decrease the negative-to-positive ion ratio.[21]

Indoors, air ion concentration is lowered by air moving through metal ducts, cigarette smoke and other air pollution, the static electricity generated by synthetic fibers, and many other human activities. Chronic ion deprivation has been associated with discomfort, lassitude, and loss of mental and physical efficiency.

Sensitivity to air ion concentrations varies widely among people. And although negative ions are often seen as "good for you," and positive ions as harmful, there are reported cases of positive ions having therapeutic effects and of life forms that are harmed by negative ions.

Awareness of air ionization and how it affects you can be valuable. But what to do about it is another matter. If you are living in a polluted city, moving to the rural mountains will probably be good for your health, and air ion concentration will be but one of the reasons why. If you are selecting a heating system, you will be better off with radiant heat than with forced air; again, the ion factor would be one of many.

Negative ion generators have been touted as the solution to air ion depletion or "pos-ion poisoning." With the proper equipment, intelligently used, they may indeed help to improve a bad situation. But irresponsible advertising and detrimental side effects also surround many of them. Potential ionizer hazards include

---

[20]"Electricity, Conduction of," *Encyclopaedia Britannica, Volume 8* (Chicago: William Benton, Publisher, 1965), p. 202.
[21]Albert P. Krueger and Sheelah Sigel, "Ions in the Air," *Human Nature*, July, 1978, pp. 46, 48.

electrical shock, production of ozone and oxides of nitrogen (both highly toxic), outgassing of plastics from warmed ionizer cases, and increased static electricity from improperly grounded units. If you choose to buy a negative ion generator, look for a dealer who has been in business for some time, check for the UL label, make a sniff test for ozone (which has a pungent odor like the fresh air after a lightning storm), and look for an ionizer with a metal case.

Air ionization is one aspect of a complex environmental picture. Krueger himself says that "The effects of ion depletion on people cannot compare with the dramatic respiratory distress caused by toxic air pollutants . . ."[22] We need to learn more about how air ions affect our health, and about which human activities improve or undermine a healthy air ion balance. I suspect that if we concentrate on healing environments in general—using appropriate building materials, lighting, heating, fresh air, delight, and so on—we will simultaneously improve the ionic environment.

Household Products

Many products used in and around buildings also contribute to the overall pollution level. Cigarette smoke tops the list, followed by so-called air fresheners, cleaning products, pesticides, laundry aids, floor and furniture waxes, aerosol sprays, paint and varnish removers, hobby materials, soft plastics, foam rubber, dry-cleaned clothes, gasoline, and personal care products such as hair spray, deodorant, nail polish, and nail polish remover.

Pesticides can be particularly troublesome, as some remain chemically active for years. They get indoors by being tracked in, by vapors coming in through open windows, and in the form of fumigation, mothballs, insecticide strips, and flea collars.

There are less harmful—and often less costly—substitutes for many of these household poisons. You can substitute a liquid or dry form of a product for an aerosol form. You can control odors by cleaning or ventilation, rather than masking them with toxic chemicals sold as air fresheners. You can purchase products designed to have low toxicity (see Resources, p. 128). You can control pests mechanically (with a fly swatter) or at their source (by

---

[22]Krueger, p. 52.

unblocking clogged pipes or draining a mud puddle). And you can replace commercial products with homemade ones. If harmful chemicals must be used, they should be used outdoors or in a well-ventilated area and stored in a sealed, fireproof compartment, preferably away from inhabited areas.

Water

We know that our health is affected by water when we drink it, but did you know that bathing or showering in it can also be hazardous? Several recent studies have found that showering in impure water for fifteen minutes can be more dangerous than drinking two liters of the same water.[23] Volatile chemicals in tap water are released into the air at faucets and showerheads, and enter our lungs as we breathe. These chemicals are also absorbed through our skin when we bathe. The skin can carry twice as much of a volatile chemical into the body as do the intestines. Volatile chemicals found in water include chlorine, chloroform, pesticides, radon, PCBs, benzene, and many others.

If you are buying land or a house, have the water supply tested before you buy. If you are not moving, check your existing water. Data on municipal water supplies are usually available from your water company, but you must also consider pollutants that enter the water via the pipes (lead from pipes and joint solder, asbestos from old asbestos-cement pipes). Though it can be expensive, you might choose to have a laboratory test the water as it comes from your faucet; check your telephone directory and get bids from several sources. Once you have a water analysis, you can tailor a filtration system to your needs. Alternatively, you can select a broad-spectrum water purifier that will protect you from a range of possible pollutants—good insurance against fluctuations in water quality.

---

[23]Julian B. Andelman, "Inhalation Exposure in the Home to Volatile Organic Contaminants of Drinking Water," *The Science of the Total Environment* (Amsterdam: Elsevier Science Publishers B.V., 1985), pp. 443-460.

CLEANING UP YOUR ENVIRONMENT

How is one to respond to this flood of indoor pollution awareness? First, reassure yourself that indoor air quality is manageable. Evaluate your own state of health as an indicator of how quickly or drastically to act. If you've been plagued by mysterious symptoms, and you suspect an environmental cause, a new sense of hope and the eventual symptomatic relief will more than compensate for any time and money you invest in clearing the air.

For most of us, Dr. Zamm has encouraging words:

> If you eat well, avoid worthless or excessive medication, choose the chemicals that you bring into your home carefully, and maintain the house sensibly, your body will probably have enough cellular energy in reserve to fight the alien chemicals and radiation you can't avoid.[24]

If your indoor pollution level or your degree of sensitivity warrant it, you can significantly improve your indoor atmosphere by revamping your ventilation system and changing interior finishes. If you plan to build a new home or other structure, designing and building for healthful indoor ecology will allow you to breathe easily. Whether as a preventive measure, or in response to an existing environmental sensitivity, you can create a milieu in which your system is not assaulted, where your body can process toxic substances it may have assimilated—where you can refresh and recharge yourself.

Builders find that "ecological construction" has much in common with solid, sensible, good-quality building. Many of the materials incorporated were in common use before the advent of synthetic building products. Your choice of materials should reflect your own chemical sensitivities, allergies, and personal tastes, as well as your climate, budget, and other design considerations. No one material or design is universally correct; as with all good design, the key is responsiveness to given conditions.

Site Selection

Many people with environmental sensitivities find that the best solution to their problems is to move to a new location.

---

[24]Zamm, p. 104.

Whether you want to create a new home, health center, or place of business, if you take health into consideration when selecting a site, you will be way ahead in providing healthful indoor air.

Evaluating a site includes everything from looking at the soil to assessing the surroundings within a ten-mile radius. Your economic circumstances, health status, and lifestyle will help you pinpoint one or more general areas where you would like to be. The next step is to learn about local weather patterns, including temperature extremes, humidity, and wind directions. Topography may also affect air movement and dissipation of potential airborne hazards. Find out about nearby land uses and pollution sources: agriculture (especially herbicide and pesticide use), forestry, industry, railroads, airports, traffic arteries, refuse disposal sites, power plants, sewage disposal facilities, and toxic waste dumps. Armed with this information, seek out a site on high ground upwind of air pollution sources. Locate your building out of the line of sight of any major power lines and microwave or broadcast towers. Avoid areas with atmospheric inversions. Ideal locations are on the shore of a large, clean body of water, in the mountains, or in the high desert.

Design

If you are creating or remodeling a building, the next step is design. Good layout and orientation are as important as material choice in determining the liveability and workability of a place. You need to look at your values, lifestyle, activities, and sensitivities, and work with givens such as solar orientation, site slope, and prevailing winds, to arrive at a healthy "fit"; Chapter 14 covers a number of general design principles for healthy places.

In designing for indoor air quality, a basic principle in the home or the workplace is to isolate and ventilate pollution-producing equipment. A detached garage will keep exhaust fumes away from the indoors. If a furnace is necessary, it can be placed in a vented room accessible only from outdoors. Office equipment, laundry machines, and cleaning and gardening chemical storage can all be confined to spaces sealed to the indoors and vented to the outdoors. Basements are best avoided, as they tend to encourage mold growth.

Building ecologically requires guessing in advance what you want to do in your home. Once you know what you want to do, it is pretty easy to design something that will let you do it—*without adversely affecting your health.*[25]

Ventilation

As we saw in the summary of the major pollutants, ventilation is a primary line of defense. For relatively low pollutant levels, well-designed ventilation may be the only measure needed. People with environmental sensitivities often find that ventilation at the source of the contaminant allows them to engage in activities that were previously harmful to them.

In tight construction, ventilation may be needed to compensate for the low rate of air exchange with the outdoors. Older buildings receive a complete exchange of fresh outdoor air for indoor air at rates of 1.5 to 3 air changes per hour due to infiltration via cracks around doors, windows, chimneys, and electrical and plumbing passageways. Newer buildings have as few as .2 to .5 air changes per hour. In light of findings about indoor air pollution, 1 to 1.5 air changes per hour are now recommended.

But tight buildings are designed to cut down on fuel bills. Do we have to choose between health and energy conservation? Not with the advent of the heat exchanger, also known as a "heat recovery ventilator" (HRV). In an HRV, thermally conditioned air on its way out of the building passes through thin-walled tubes of metal or paper that interfinger with incoming-air tubes. The desired heat can thus be transferred from the exhaust air to the fresh incoming air, recovering some of the investment made in heating it. The thermal exchange is not total, but HRVs can recover 60% to 85% of the heat from exhaust air,[26] while constantly diluting contaminants in the indoor air. Heat exchangers are most effective where air exchange rates are lowest, gaseous pollutant levels are highest, and the difference between indoor and outdoor temperature is greatest. An HRV system should be professionally designed

---

[25]Bruce M. Small, "Creating Your Own Safe Environment," *Environ*, Fall, 1985, p. 6.
[26]Suzanne and Ed Randegger, "HRVs Help Reduce Home Pollution," *Environ*, Fall-Winter, 1986-87, p. 19.

and installed to ensure proper equipment selection, sizing, and layout.

Whatever form of ventilation you use, venting a pollutant at its source can reduce the overall ventilation rate required and can make a wider range of activities available to the chemically sensitive. Stove hood vents and fireplace chimneys are typical examples of source ventilation, but indoor health researcher Bruce Small has taken the principle even further. He has designed ways of fully surrounding and venting pollution-causing items in the home,

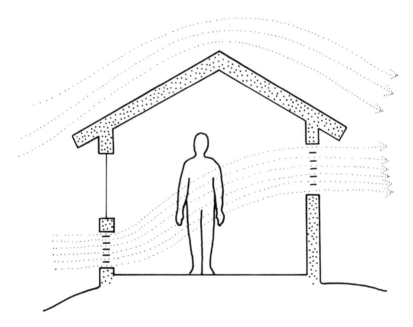

making their use more tolerable. For example, a person who is sensitive to the trace odors of plastic electronic chips and capacitors and burning dust that rise from the back of a television set can enclose that television in a cabinet that has a glass door and a vent or duct to the outside. Hobby and workshop materials, as well as work clothes, can be kept in a vented closet. Cooking appliances can be grouped along one wall for easier venting.

Some basic rules apply to any ventilation system. Be sure that all combustion appliances (furnace, water heater) have their own air supply and exhaust outlet. Locate air intakes carefully to avoid drawing in exhaust air from your own building, other buildings, or passing automobiles. Guard against insulation or other fibrous materials entering a duct system and being combined with indoor air, and check ducts regularly for microbial growth.

Filtration

Filtration can increase the effectiveness of any ventilation system. Incoming air can be filtered to remove pollen and other particles. Recirculated air can be cleansed of certain pollutants as it passes through filters. However, if filters are not cleaned or replaced at appropriate intervals, they can harbor bacteria and reintroduce pollutants to the air, creating more problems than they solve.

You might use only one of the variety of filters available, or you might use several in series. Physical or mechanical filtration involves fibrous filters and removes particles such as dust and pollen from the air; the larger particles are most effectively removed. Activated carbon and other chemical filters remove many organic vapors and some inorganic ones, including ozone, carbon monoxide, and nitrogen dioxide; some carbon filters are specially impregnated to remove formaldehyde from the air. Electrostatic filters remove dust, pollen, and smaller particles from the air; "passive" electrostatic filters are preferable to other types, which can generate ozone. Sensitive people should investigate any filter for components that may produce reactions. Filtration systems should always be designed to handle effectively the types and volume of pollutants that you wish to remove from your indoor air.

BUILDING MATERIALS

Of course, the fewer pollutants you introduce indoors, the less ventilation and filtration you will need. Mary Oetzel, a low-toxic building materials consultant, says that for the general public, "if we can reduce the chemical load in a house by maybe 50% to 60%, we're doing a good job;" for the highly sensitive she recommends reducing the load by 80% or 95%.[27] Whether you are

---

[27]Debra Lynn Dadd, "Less-Toxic Building Materials, An Interview With Mary Oetzel," *Everything Natural*, September/October, 1986, p. 16.

modifying an existing building, constructing a new building, or searching for a building to inhabit, knowledge about non-toxic building materials can help you avoid costly mistakes.

Designer-builder Paul Bierman-Lytle says, "We know that natural, healthy products do more than make you feel good, they actually enhance your living and working spaces, improve your productivity, and calm and refresh your spirit."[28]

Structure

If you are building a new room or a new building, choose structural materials to fit your sensitivities. Many people appear unaffected by standard wood framing, but if you are sensitive to softwood outgassing or mold (which can thrive on wood), you may prefer to investigate other materials. As an inert material, steel framing is the first choice of some sensitive people. Since the steel members arrive coated with petroleum products, they should be washed before being assembled. Concrete and masonry (concrete block, brick, stone) can be "safe" materials if they do not emit radon, if the concrete mix doesn't include toxic additives, and if mold growth is avoided. Other earth materials such as adobe, rammed earth, and clay are well received by many environmentally sensitive people and have a warmer feeling than does concrete.

Insulation

Insulation, if sealed inside a cavity wall, is rarely harmful to most people. However, many insulations can cause health damage if they are installed carelessly, introducing particles, fibers, or gasses into the airstream or skin pores of installers or inhabitants.

The insulations generally preferred for a "healthy" building are: Air-Krete, a cementitious, foamed-in product; cotton batts; and foil-faced bubble pack (see Resources, p. 126). Foil-faced fiberglass batts and blown-in fiberglass are also acceptable if properly installed—but breathing in loose fibers can cause health damage. Some sensitive people also react to the resins in batts or to asphalt

---

[28]Debra Lynn Dadd, "The All-Natural House, An Interview With Paul Bierman-Lytle," *Everything Natural,* September/October, 1986, p. 13.

emulsion on draft paper-faced batts. Rock wool sometimes contains lignite or mineral oil, which might not be tolerated by some dwellers.

Plant materials such as straw and cork are getting renewed attention as insulating materials, as many people are looking for more "natural" products, but some cork has a strong smell.

Vermiculite and perlite are natural products low in toxicity, but they are only advised for use in masonry cavities that are permanently sealed. Otherwise, breathing their finer particles can cause the lung disease "silicosis."[29]

Rigid foams (polystyrene, polyurethane polyisocyanurate, and phenolic) release toxic fumes when burned and should probably only be used on the exterior or masonry walls.

Blown-in cellulosic insulation is made from old newspapers impregnated with fire-retardant chemicals. Some people have had adverse reactions to the newsprint, ink, chemical treatment, or dust particles of cellulose insulation.

Urea-formaldehyde foam insulation has already been discussed (see p. 103); avoid it in existing buildings, and don't use it in new ones.

Floors

The ideal floor material generates no gasses or airborne particles, needs no wax or other toxic finishes, is easily cleaned of dust, and holds little or no electrical charge.

Concrete provides the most inert floor material—again, if not radon-emitting. It can be colored and textured or patterned while wet to resemble tile or stone. Since concrete is porous, it needs to be sealed. A sealer should be chosen carefully to avoid adding harmful chemicals to the air. Concrete floors and radiant heating tubes make a good team (see Chapter 9). When using a radiant heated slab, it is best to avoid floor coverings, especially if they are glued down; the heat can volatilize the adhesive and the floor covering, producing fumes for years.

Soil-cement floors have a warmer "feel" than concrete and

---

[29]Zamm, p. 149.

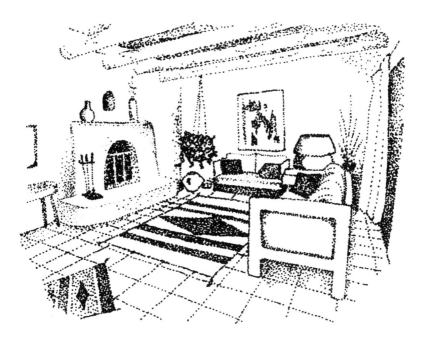

are not as hard. They, too, can be pressed to simulate tile and can be paired with radiant heating.

Another low-toxic floor material is hardwood nailed to an acceptable subfloor (such as tongue-and-groove pine decking or exterior-grade plywood). Hardwood also requires a finish, which should be selected carefully. A growing number of low-toxic products are available; some even specifically formulated to be tolerable to the chemically sensitive. Polyurethane can be appropriate because it outgasses quickly and doesn't require waxing. It should, however, be applied in warm weather with good ventilation; residents are advised to go on vacation while polyurethane is being applied. Another solution is to buy pre-finished wood flooring if sensitivities allow. (See Resources, p. 128, for sources of other low-toxicity wood finishes).

Nonporous ceramic tile is often recommended for "clean" floors and walls, but some basic principles must be observed to avoid introducing problems. It is best to apply tile on concrete or masonry surfaces. Tile should be set in a thick mortar bed or with "thin-set" cement, but not applied with toxic adhesives. Avoid offensive chemicals in the mortar or grout, such as epoxies, furans, and organic mastics. The grout joints between tiles are notorious for mold growth. This can be discouraged by keeping joints narrow, using larger tiles to make joints less frequent, leaving the grout flush with the surface of the tile rather than concave, and keeping the area as dry as possible. Grout can be sealed with water glass (sodium silicate) or beeswax.

Terrazzo, a material made of stone chips in a cement base and then polished, is preferred by many people. It can either be poured and polished in place or purchased in precast units. It requires sealing and waxing, and so shouldn't be used by people sensitive to such products.

Wall-to-wall carpeting is generally not recommended. It generates dust and vapors, traps house dust which is stirred up by walking on it, harbors mold if damp, is often delivered permeated with insecticides, and can generate a static charge when walked on. When adhesives and/or rubberoid paddings are used in carpet installation, they create additional hazards by outgassing. Area rugs that can be removed for cleaning (without toxic chemicals!)—especially washable cotton throw rugs—are highly preferred.

Walls

Gypsum plaster is the material of choice for covering interior walls. It can be trowelled over a plaster board lath, and dries to a hard, white, chemically stable surface. It can be the final wall surface as is. If plain white walls are undesirable, tints can be added to the wet plaster before application.

Hardwood panelling (birch, oak, walnut, ash, hickory, maple, beech, cherry, or teak) is not universally recommended, but it can be an excellent wall finish for someone not sensitive to hardwoods. The wood should be nailed, not glued, to the wall.

Brick, tile, stone, and stucco are excellent wall materials for many people. Similar care should be taken when installing brick or stone as when setting tile (see pp. 122-3).

Standard gypsum wallboard is acceptable to many people, but some react to the paper binder on some brands of wallboard. The compound typically used for sealing joints between the boards contains hazardous chemicals, but it can be replaced with trowelled plaster. The biggest drawback to gypsum board is that it needs to be painted or wallpapered.

Paints in general are now less toxic than they were several years ago. Lead and mercury have been removed and volatile organic compounds reduced. But most standard paint types are somewhat-to-very toxic until they are fully cured—a process which can take many months. Some companies now offer low-toxic paints especially formulated for the chemically sensitive. And several brands of plant-based paint are available; their smell is very pleasant to some, but too strong for others. Casein paints rarely pose a problem in themselves, but their milk base makes them susceptible to mold growth in damp areas (see Resources, p. 126).

Before using a particular paint, you can test it for tolerability. One method is to coat a piece of wood with the paint to be tested; when it is thoroughly dry, place it inside your pillowcase, on top of the pillow, where your nostrils will be exposed to it. After a night of sleeping with the paint, you'll know whether you can live with it. Another method is to place a small quantity of paint (or any other substance you wish to test) in a glass jar and leave it in the sunlight for several hours. Then open the jar, sniff the contents, and observe your reactions. Be cautious!

Wallpaper is not recommended. The paper itself outgasses inks and paints and may contribute cellulose particles to the air. Wallpaper paste typically contains harmful chemicals; homemade pastes may encourage mold growth.

Other potentially harmful wall materials are pressed wood panels, cork bound with petrochemicals, and vinyl sheets or tiles. Vinyl is inappropriate both because of its own outgassing and because of the noxious adhesives used in applying it.

THE OASIS

Environmentally sensitive people who live or work with others or in areas that receive mild contamination will benefit from establishing one room as an "oasis" for themselves. At home, it might be a bedroom or study. At work, it could be a private office. Seal off the oasis from other areas, and scrupulously examine and test every item or material installed in the room. Filter incoming air meticulously. The object is to create one place—a haven—where the sensitive person can retreat regularly from the constant irritants outside, allowing the body to relax, process toxic substances, and recharge itself without threats. A person thus recharged is often able to function normally in the "outside" world. In fact, sometimes it is sufficient to construct or remodel a single-room oasis, rather than remodel or construct a whole building. An oasis might also be the first step for someone planning a new building; it serves as a testing ground for appropriate materials and appliances.

RESOURCES

Books

The Body Electric: Electromagnetism and the Foundation of Life, by Robert O. Becker, M.D. (William Morrow, 1985).

Clean & Green: The Complete Guide to Nontoxic and Environmentally Safe Housekeeping, by Annie Berthold-Bond (Ceres Press, 1991).

Cross Currents: The Perils of Electropollution, The Promise of Electromedicine, by Robert O. Becker, M.D. (Jeremy P. Tarcher, Inc., 1990).

Currents of Death, by Paul Brodeur (Simon & Schuster, 1989).

Ecological Architecture, by Richard L. Crowther (Butterworth Architecture, 80 Montvale Ave., Stoneham, MA 02180, 1992).

Environmental Quality in Offices, by Jacqueline C. Vischer (Van Nostrand Reinhold, 1988).

Health and Light, by John N. Ott (Devin-Adair, 1973).

Healthful Houses: How to Design & Build Your Own, by Clint Good & Debra Dadd (Guaranty Press, 1988).

Healthy Building for a Better Earth, (Trust for the Future, 2704 12th Ave. S., Nashville, TN 37204, 1991).

The Healthy Home, by Linda Mason Hunter (Rodale Press, 1989).

The Healthy House, by John Bower (Lyle Stuart, 1989).

Healthy House Building: A Design & Construction Guide, by John Bower (7471 Shiloh Rd., Unionville, IN 47468, 1993).

Interior Concerns Resource Guide, by Victoria Schomer (P.O. Box 2386, Mill Valley, CA 94942).

The Natural Formula Book for Home and Yard, edited by Dan Wallace (Rodale Press, 1982).

The Natural House Book, by David Pearson (Simon & Schuster, 1989).

The Nontoxic Home & Office, by Debra Lynn Dadd (Jeremy P. Tarcher, 1992).

Nontoxic, Natural, and Earthwise, by Debra Lynn Dadd (Jeremy P. Tarcher, 1990).

Places of the Soul, by Christopher Day (The Aquarian Press, 1990).

Radon: The Invisible Threat, by Michael Lafavore (Rodale Press, 1987).

Safe Home Resource Guide, by Lloyd Publishing (24 East Ave., Suite 1300, New Canaan, CT 06840).

Toxic Carpet III, by Glenn Beebe (P.O. Box 399086, Cincinnati, OH 45239, 1991).

Your Home, Your Health, and Well-Being, by David Rousseau (Ten Speed Press, 1988).

Periodicals

Building with Nature, P.O. Box 369, Gualala, CA 95445.

Environ: A Magazine for Ecologic Living, P.O. Box 2204, Fort Collins, CO 80522.

Environmental Building News, RR1 Box 161, Brattleboro, VT 05301.

Environmental Resource Guide, 9 Jay Gould Ct., P.O. Box 753, Waldorf, MD 20604.

Green Alternatives, 38 Montgomery St., Rhinebeck, NY 12572.

IBE Newsletter, International Institute for Bau-Biologie & Ecology, Inc., Box 387, Clearwater, FL 34615.

Indoor Air Bulletin, P.O. Box 8446, Santa Cruz, CA 95061-8446.

Indoor Air Review, 5335 Wisconsin Ave. NW, Suite 440, Washington, D.C. 20015.

Interior Concerns Newsletter, P.O. Box 2386, Mill Valley, CA 94942.

The New Reactor, Environmental Health Network of California, P.O. Box 1155, Larkspur, CA 94977.

General

Environmental Construction Outfitters, 44 Crosby St., New York, NY 10012, (800) 238-5008.

Healthful Hardware, P.O. Box 3217, Prescott, AZ 86303, (602) 445-8225.

The Living Source, 7005 Woodway Dr., #214, Waco, TX 76712, (817) 776-4878.

N.E.E.D.S., 527 Charles Avenue, 12-A, Syracuse, NY 13209, (800) 634-1380.

Nontoxic Environments, 9392 S. Gribble Rd., Canby, OR 97013, (503) 266-5244.

Insulation

Air Krete, Inc., P.O. Box 380, Weedsport, NY 13166, (315) 834-6609.

Cotton Unlimited, Inc. (InsulCot), P.O. Box 760, Post, TX 79356, (806) 495-3511.

Insul-Tray (cardboard sleeves for cellulose insulation), E. 1881 Crestview Dr., Shelton, WA 98584, (206) 427-5930.

Out on Bale (un)Ltd. (information on straw), 1037 E. Linden St., Tucson, AZ 85719, (602) 624-1673.

Perlite Institute, Inc., 88 New Dorp Plaza, Staten Island, NY 10306, (718) 351-5723.

Rector Mineral Trading Corp. (cork), 9 West Prospect Ave., Mount Vernon, NY 10550, (914) 699-5755.

Reflectix, Inc. (foil-faced bubble-pack type), P.O. Box 108, Markleville, IN 46056, (800) 879-3645.

Fabrics

The Cotton Place, P.O. Box 59721, Dallas, TX 75229, (214) 243-4149.

Dona Designs, 825 Northlake Drive, Richardson, TX 75080, (214) 235-0485.

Homespun Fabrics, P.O. Box 3223, Ventura, CA 93003, (805) 642-8111.

Jantz Design (bedding/furnishings), P.O. Box 3071, Santa Rosa, CA 95402, (707) 823-8834, (800) 365-6563.

Testfabrics, P.O. Box 420, Middlesex, NJ 08846, (908) 469-6446.

Paints, Sealers, Finishes

AFM Enterprises, Inc., 1140 Stacy Court, Riverside, CA 92507, (714) 781-6860.

Auro Products, Sinan Company, P.O. Box 857, Davis, CA 95617-0857, (916) 753-3104.

BIOFA Products, BAU, Inc., P.O. Box 190, Alton, NH 03809, (603) 364-2400.

Eco Designs, 1365 Rufina Circle, Santa Fe, NM 87501, (800) 621-2591.

Miller Paint Company, 317 SE Grand Avenue, Portland, OR 97214, (503) 233-4021.

Murco Wall Products, 300 NE 21st Street, Fort Worth, TX 76106, (817) 626-1987.

Nigra Enterprises, 5699 Kanan Road, Agoura CA 91301, (818) 889-6877.

The Old-Fashioned Milk Paint Company, P.O. Box 222, Groton, MA, 01450, (508) 448-6336.

Pace Chem Industries, Inc., 779 S. La Grange Ave., Newbury Park, CA 91320, (805) 499-2911.

Floor Coverings

Hendricksen Naturlich, 6761 Sebastopol Ave., Sebastopol, CA 95472, (707) 829-3989.

Forbo Industries, Humboldt Industrial Park, Maplewood Dr., P.O. Box 667, Hazleton, PA 18201, (800) 233-0475.

· CHAPTER · 12 ·

Plants and Gardens

Hope never dies in a real gardener's heart.

—DR. C. F. MENNINGER

Relationships with plants provide a powerful ongoing connection with life. Though they are not part of a building, strictly speaking, they have an important role in the built environment, and they may be just what we need to overcome some of the isolating effects of buildings. Simply gazing upon a plant can lift the spirits and calm the mind. To care for plants releases us from our mental ruts, physical tensions, and sense of alienation; we become meaningful to our plants' flourishing, as they do to ours. The presence of plants can also modulate our indoor atmosphere, influencing temperature, humidity, and air quality.

In a rural environment, indoor plants can visually and functionally bring the outdoors in. In an urban environment, plants can reconnect us with the earth and life's cycles. Horticulturist Elvin McDonald underscores this notion:

> I work hard a lot, I play hard less than I would like. It's not easy to make ends meet, to work against deadlines, and to keep calm.
> But I am calm most of the time, thanks to my day-to-day involvement with plants. Sometimes all I need to feel peaceful is to touch a velvety petal or furry leaf or to remove the withered flowers from the African violets.[1]

Introducing abundant indoor plants is one of the easiest ways to transform your living and working environments. Their presence is both calming and enlivening. They are constantly changing,

---

[1]Elvin McDonald, *Plants as Therapy* (New York: Praeger Publishers, 1976), p. 5.

responding to their inner rhythms, planetary cycles, and the care you give them. Plants can augment any design theme you choose, from refined and controlled to a primal jungle. Plants may even improve your social life (an important element of health); Elvin McDonald believes that people relax and linger in a room full of plants.

Nancy Jack Todd and John Todd of the New Alchemy Institute, an ecological research organization, firmly believe in the health benefits of plants:

> The enjoyment to be found in the air of a forest or a meadow breeze is not illusory. Vegetation interacts rapidly and efficiently with flowing air to improve its quality and smell, and these beneficial natural processes can be duplicated indoors. Placing clusters of plants near a window is an effective and simple ecological solution. The plants breathe during the day, giving off fresh oxygen and purifying the air.[2]

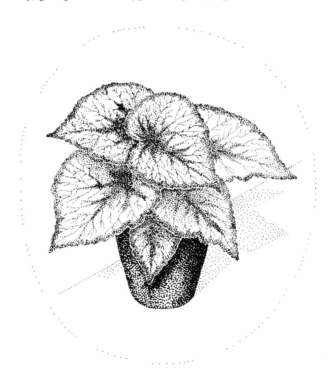

---

[2]Nancy Jack Todd and John Todd, *Bioshelters, Ocean Arks, City Farming: Ecology as the Basis of Design* (San Francisco: Sierra Club Books, 1984), p. 110.

Similarly, indoor plant consultant Louise Odiorne believes that it is important to establish "Human Climate" via the "Indoor Eden Effect".[3]

> This means that the same life supportive, symbiotic relationship is set up within a building as exists outside between plants and animals (people). We have evolved, since the Garden of Eden, within these conditions of oxygen-carbon dioxide-moisture exchange brought about and controlled by living plants. So why not arrange to let this process continue to support us within the shelter we build for ourselves in any climate on earth?[4]

Involvement with plants can be healing in other ways, as the successes of horticultural therapy demonstrate. Horticultural therapy is used in treating a wide range of physical and mental disabilities; people of every age, illness, or therapeutic need can participate in some aspect of plant care. Dr. Howard A. Rusk, Director of the Institute of Rehabilitation Medicine, New York University Medical Center, describes some of the psychological aspects of horticultural therapy:

> Some patients are difficult to reach and motivate. Working with plants may provide an impetus and initiate a response. Something as simple as the growth of roots on a cutting suspended in a glass of water, or a bud preparing to open, may provide the key. One of the great advantages of gardening is that it is not a static activity. There is always something happening—a new sprout, shoot, or leaf is forming, a flower is opening or fading and has to be removed. Then the cycle begins all over again. Most important, especially for patients who are totally dependent on others for assistance in even the smallest tasks, is a living thing depending on them for care and sustenance. This gives the patient the will to go on and an interest in the future.[5]

The National Council for Therapy and Rehabilitation Through Horticulture (NCTRH) in Mt. Vernon, Virginia has hundreds of success stories on file. One tells of a group of ten women at a state institution for the emotionally disturbed who had been given up as hopeless. "Soon after an introduction to plant therapy they walked almost half a mile to the greenhouse and everyone talked sensibly. Eight of the women went home

---

[3]"Human Climate" and "Indoor Eden Effect" © 1969 by Louise Odiorne.
[4]Louise Odiorne, personal correspondence to Carol Venolia, 1973.
[5]*Ibid.*, p. 112.

within two months; the other two did not have a home to go to."[6] In another testimonial, a former prison warden said that horticultural therapy was the only means by which he had been able to rehabilitate some of the toughest criminals.

Robert Steffen, farm manager for a boys' home, observes:

> Gardening is good therapy for young and old. The earth has great healing power. It is the plant, of course, which makes it all possible. Simply realizing that we could not exist on this planet without the plant should be significant. . . . Plants are indeed a source of great hope for our time and for the many people who are disturbed, frustrated, and concerned about the future. Knowing and understanding plants can give them hope and reassurance that with death there follows life, and the great cycles of the seasons are part of even greater rhythms of the universe that are not dependent on mortal man's manipulation.[7]

If the severely disturbed can receive such sustenance by caring for plants, why not others? Elvin McDonald finds that business people who have a collection of healthy, well-groomed plants in their offices are usually calmer, more efficient, and easier to deal with than those who don't have plants or whose plants are neglected.

No one need deny themselves plants. Even in a small, dark apartment, lighting and love can produce an abundant garden. With an operable window, window box planters can enliven the vista from indoors and enhance the building's appearance from outdoors. If there's a balcony or deck, it can be transformed from a barren place into a lush food- and flower-producing paradise. And if you have a yard, the sky's the limit.

The outdoor garden is a transition zone between the private, secure world of the indoors and the larger realm of nature and civilization. The garden is a place where we can be at home in a spot of our creation and yet be in communion with sun, wind, rain, and the mysteries of growth. We work in concert with the forces of nature to help a garden flourish. Through the cycles of plant growth we are linked to the seasons and to change. Gardening is also an excellent way to get daily sunshine and exercise while

---

[6]McDonald, p. 109.
[7]*Ibid.*, p. 80.

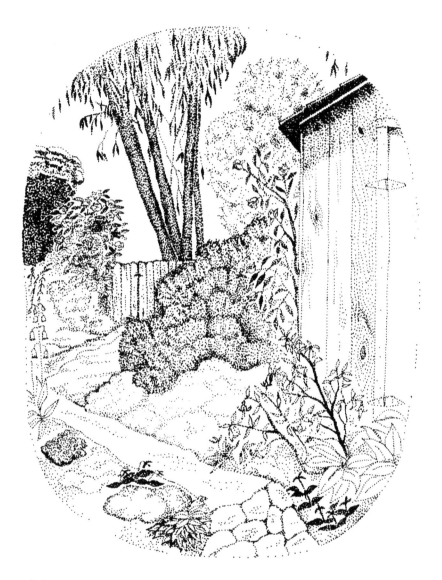

doing something enjoyable and productive—much more interesting than jogging on a treadmill!

By arranging outdoor plants knowledgeably, we can use them to temper our environment in gentle ways: a deciduous tree or vine on the south side of a yard or building will provide cooling summer shade and admit warm winter sun; a dense planting belt can deflect unwanted noise or provide protection from the wind; and ground covers, shrubs, and trees can reduce irritating reflection and glare.

The garden also provides an opportunity to be in direct contact with the earth—something that rarely happens inside modern buildings. We seem to be missing something essential—perhaps a rooted feeling—when we don't stand barefoot on the ground from time to time. A gardener friend of mine suggested that a crucial element in a healing garden is a clean, smooth, earthen path for barefoot walking.

In a garden, not only can you have relationships with myriad plants, but you can also provide habitats for birds, butterflies, frogs, squirrels, and countless other animals that can enrich your visual and sonic environment. Even in the city you can create a small wildlife sanctuary, making an environment that is healing to you, to the animals that are drawn to it, and, in a small but significant way, to the city itself. The National Wildlife Federation, through its Backyard Wildlife Habitat program, provides guidelines for starting your own wildlife sanctuary.[8] Chapter 10 of this book includes suggestions for attracting birds to your garden.

Gardens are not completely free of health hazards, however. For the allergic, it is best to be tested and possibly treated for specific pollen allergies and to avoid using irritating plants. Ponds can be lovely to look at, but if they are stagnant they can be breeding grounds for insects and for molds which will release spores into the air. If toxic chemicals are used to control insects or weeds, they can easily be inhaled or ingested, resulting in everything from minor irritation to cancer. But with proper precautions, the health benefits of the garden will far outweigh the risks.

Buildings designed to relate closely to gardens can be exceptionally satisfying environments. When building and garden are shaped in concert, each augments the other. Windows can be placed for garden views from a desk, a bathtub, or a social area. Building forms can create microclimates to protect plants in courtyards, atriums, or sunny corners. Some enlightened corporations

---

[8]For information write to: Backyard Wildlife Habitat Program, Dept. 122, National Wildlife Federation, 1412 Sixteenth Street, N.W., Washington, D.C. 20036.

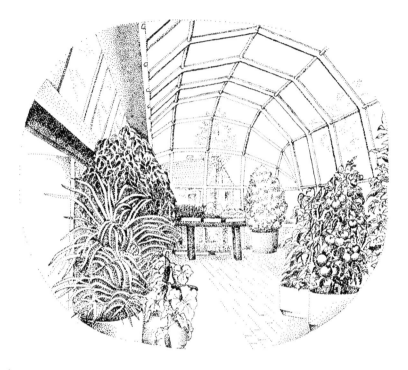

have found that gardens visible from work areas improve employee morale and productivity.

Whether in a window-sized greenhouse or on an outdoor acre, the significance of food gardening cannot be overemphasized. As mentioned in the discussion of kitchens and nourishment (see Chapter 13), by growing our own food we begin to recall what many of us have forgotten: that we participate in a complex system of interdependent natural cycles.

> Parks, street trees, and manicured lawns do very little to establish the connection between us and the land. They teach us nothing of its productivity, nothing of its capacities. Many people who are born, raised, and live out their lives in cities simply do not know where the food they eat comes from or what a living garden is like. Their only connection with the productivity of the land comes from the packaged tomatoes on the supermarket shelf. But contact with the land and its growing process is not simply a quaint nicety from the past that we can let go of casually. More likely, it is a basic part of the process of organic security.[9]

---

[9]Christopher Alexander, *A Pattern Language* (New York: Oxford University Press, 1977), p. 820.

Along similar lines, designer Day Chahroudi suggests that people live in "Biospheres"—"an integration of a house, a greenhouse, a solar heater, and a solar still."

> By making a living area more self-sustaining, a lot of long distorted communications loops are replaced by short accurate loops. Instead of working at a job unrelated to tomatoes, getting paid and buying tomatoes from someone who never met the people who grow the tomatoes, if you live in a biosphere and you want to eat a tomato, you grow a tomato.[10]

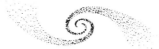

Close your eyes and imagine that you are in your favorite landscape. It can be a place where you've been, a place you've heard of, or a fantasy creation. Notice how the air feels: is it warm or cool, moist or dry, moving or still? Are there any sounds—birds, crickets, wind, moving water, other people? What kinds of smells are there? What is the landscape like: is it wide open, dense with growth, on a boundary between forest and meadow? Is the setting wild, cultivated, or some of both? What land forms do you see? What kinds of plants are there—flowers, trees, shrubs, vines, vegetables, fruit? Are animals present? Other people? Is there water in this landscape? What are you standing or sitting on? What do you like to do in this place? Walk around in this imaginary place; do some areas have special qualities or feelings? Look around and notice which features give the place its appealing character.

Now keep the feeling or image of your imaginary place, and return to your present environment. Does anything around you correspond with the imagined place—the quality of light, the temperature, the open or closed feeling? Can you alter a few features to bring your current environment more into harmony with the one you envisioned? Which elements will go farthest symbolically or actually to bring the qualities of your fantasy place into your life? You don't need to recreate the African savanna or Amazon jungle in your city apartment or suburban backyard, but if introducing a few evocative plants and other elements brings you some peace of mind, it's well worth it.

---

[10]Day Chahroudi, "Biosphere," *Mother Earth News*, December, 1972, center poster.

· III ·

·S·Y·N·T·H·E·S·I·S·

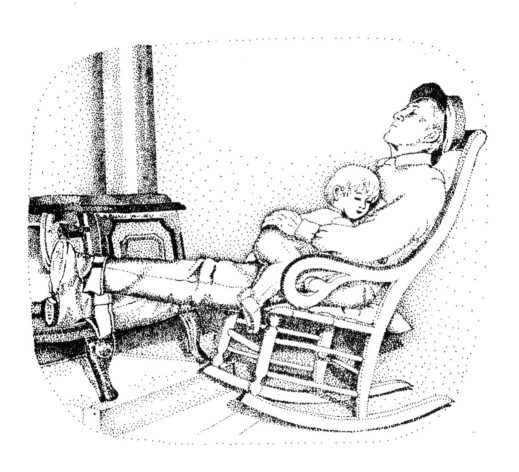

· CHAPTER · 13 ·

Applications

*. . . rest assured, anything that relaxes the body, stimulates the
mind, and refreshes the spirit is healing.*

—BETTY WOOD

In Section II, each chapter examined a different aspect of our built
environment. Though focusing on parts of the picture allows us
to develop our understanding, we need to re-integrate those pieces
into the whole; to do otherwise would be to miss the point entirely. We respond to the whole environment—to the balance, interactions, and integration of all the parts. For every activity we
engage in, we can create a place where symbol, light, color,
warmth, sound, air, and planting contribute to the healthfulness
of that activity.

SLEEP

We know that the quality of a night's sleep can determine the
character of the whole next day. We know that we spend a third
of our time asleep in bed. We also know that a good night's sleep
and an undisturbed dream pattern are essential to our well-being
and mental health. And yet most of us pay little attention to the
environment of sleep as such. After all, when we're sleeping, we're
"unconscious," "somewhere else."

> Are bedrooms empty places, or gateways to deeper realms of experience?
> Does consciousness drift away here or is this its temple?[1]

---

[1]Curt Lamb, *Homestyles* (New York: St. Martin's Press, 1979), p. 29.

When we sleep, our breathing rhythm changes, our brain waves take on characteristic sleep and dreaming patterns, our vision moves from an external to an internal focus, our body temperature is altered, our motor responses are lessened, and our hearing and smelling abilities go essentially unchanged. In a sense, we become different design clients as sleepers than when awake.

The typical bedroom, however, represents a minimal response to this rich time. The room is usually a catch-all for multiple functions; it serves as sleeping room, dressing area, personal library, sexual retreat, office, playroom, sickroom, storage place, and often an individual's only private space within a home. If we break out of our standard view of the bedroom and look at how each activity is best accommodated, we can usually find more satisfying solutions without necessarily taking up any more floor space.

The place where we sleep molds our sleeping experience in ways both direct and indirect. A look at our physiological and

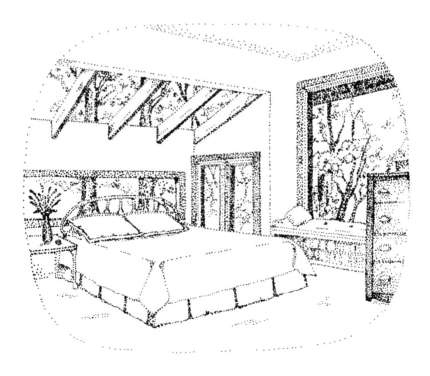

psychological needs before, during, and after sleep can help us craft a place that honors the central role sleep plays in our lives. By freeing ourselves for healthy, natural sleep, we allow our dreams to fulfill their rightful role in our overall health as well. Ancient Greeks were masters at "dream incubation"; popular rural healing temples were devoted to the belief that healing messages would be delivered in dreams to the properly prepared (see Chapter 15).

During sleep, the difference between our body's core temperature and shell temperature is reduced, lessening our adaptability to external temperature change. If we are either too warm or too cool, our sleep is disturbed. Cold-weather thermal comfort in bed depends more on the temperature at the body under the covers than in the room at large. In the ideal situation, the skin is well insulated and the air is slightly cool. The recommended air temperature is 60° to 65°F.[2] If blankets weigh more than a total of seven pounds, their weight will also disturb sleep; in cold climates a fluffy comforter is a good choice. Electric blankets, mattress warmers, and electrically heated water beds may be harmful because they set up an unfamiliar electric field. According to the Electric Power Research Institute, pregnant women who sleep under electric blankets—even if they are plugged in but not turned on—may be at greater-than-average risk for miscarriages.[3] If the bed must be prewarmed, try a hot water bottle, or take a hot bath and then jump in between a down comforter and a lambswool mattress cover (or whatever materials your allergies allow).

Wherever possible the sleeping environment should include fresh air. The time-honored advice of sleeping with the window open is still good. Airing the sleeping room thoroughly before going to bed helps even more. Mahatma Gandhi slept outdoors, amazed that people chose to inhale the "poisoned air" they and their companions exhaled.[4] In this country, the turn-of-the-century sleeping porches allowed sleepers the benefits of abundant

---

[2]Fanger, *Indoor Climate*, p. 763.

[3]From *Earth Island Journal*, summarized in *Everything Natural*, July/August, 1987, p. 6.

[4]Mariane Kohler, *101 Recipes for Sound Sleep* (New York: Walker and Company, 1965), p. 37.

fresh air without allowing it to invade the thermal space of the rest of the house.

Under some circumstances, fresh air is not the best choice: some people with allergies or weather sensitivities are better protected from outside air; infants, the ill, and the elderly don't tolerate cold air as well as the general population. If you do sleep with closed windows and heated air, take extra precautions to ensure that the air contains some moisture. Otherwise, you risk sleeping badly and waking up with a dry, sore throat.

Noise is as much of an issue when we're asleep as when we're awake. Loud noises are fairly obvious; they awaken us, jolting us from restful sleep. But the lower-level sounds (30 to 50db) can be even more harmful; sounds not quite loud enough to awaken us nevertheless cause us to shift from deep to light sleep. While we may believe that we adapt to nighttime noise, studies show that our bodies never habituate to it; we are denied the benefits of normal sleep, our energy levels and efficiency are impaired, and serious long-term effects may result. (See Chapter 10 for noise-reduction techniques).

By the same token, soothing music or nature sounds can be a positive element in the sleep environment. Before sleep, relaxing music helps to calm the body and mind and can mask irritating noises. One author suggests peaceful music during sleep, even if it is not consciously heard, because it encourages pleasant dreams. But loud, insistent music with lots of percussion can produce nightmares.[5] If you live in an area where an open window admits the sounds of nature, they, too, may be conducive to sleep. Wind in tree branches, breaking waves, rain, or the sound of a brook may lull you to sleep (see Chapter 10).

> The sounds of nature, when we are safely shut up indoors, reinforce our feeling of security. . . . Sleep is associated with a feeling of security.[6]

Though we rarely think about it, our sense of smell also contributes to our sleep experience. Unpleasant odors or stale-smelling air is not only disruptive in itself but usually indicates unhealthful conditions that need attention. But we can also use

---

[5]*Ibid.*, p. 133.
[6]*Ibid.*, p. 39.

scent to improve our sleep. Lavender is the best scent, but orange blossom, heliotrope, oil of bergamot, and essence of benzoin are also good sleep-inducing scents. You can rub them on yourself, scent your sheets with them, or put several drops in a bowl of water to gently fill the air. Of course, if you have any allergies, such scents should be carefully tested or avoided altogether.

Color may affect the nature of our sleep, even with our eyes closed. As mentioned in Chapter 8, some experiments have shown that blind or blindfolded people are able to detect color differences. Color healers believe strongly in choosing the right colors for bedrooms and bedding. Blues and greens are often suggested for their relaxing qualities. Pink sheets are said to encourage loving feelings.

The visual impact of the area also plays an important role in our sleep. What you gaze upon before you fall asleep, and what you see when you first wake up, can enhance or undermine a good night's sleep. Ideally, before sleep we would see a serene environment that induces feelings of lightness, security, and coziness: warm, low lighting, soothing colors, and soft textures. We won't be helped by seeing clutter, unfinished projects, or anything disruptive, distracting, or agitating. I would never put my desk in the same room with my bed; when I'm on my way to sleep, I don't want reminders of mental activity, writing, bill-paying, and the like.

Bedroom lighting should be soft, warm, and relaxing. For bedtime reading, a single brighter light in the right place will create an appropriate focus. If you like moonlight, a properly located window or skylight will let you fall asleep to its romantic glow.

In the morning, the way we awaken sets the tone for our whole day. A loud alarm invading your sleep is inhumane and will more often than not interrupt a crucial sleep phase. Allowing the morning sunlight to awaken you (not by shining directly in your eyes) is ideal; the gradual increase in light and warmth will allow your body to complete its brainwave cycle, and you can awaken with your biological clock attuned by the rising sun as it was meant to be. A gradual awakening in pleasant, cozy surroundings will allow you to reflect on your dreams, bid them farewell, and contemplate the day ahead with positive feelings. Think about what colors, textures, forms, spaces, and objects you would like to see upon awakening—things that would validate your night's journey and bring the new day to you in an unthreatening way.

We all have rituals that precede going to bed and follow getting out of bed. Usually we are barely conscious of them as such, or of their role in our healthful sleep. But if you begin to contemplate these rituals and then think of ways to accommodate them so that they can increase your bedtime or waking serenity, your life will have a greater feeling of wholeness. Bathing, quiet conversation, grooming, undressing and dressing, meditating, reading, eating, and other activities are all part of the sleep-transition experience. If you like to read before or after sleep, but have no comfortable place to do so—no convenient spot for your books, no appropriate reading light—you're more likely to build up stress than to release it. If you have to run all over the house to brush your teeth, undress, read, turn out lights, and jump in bed, you may be more scattered than centered when you hit the sheets. Think of ways to arrange and augment your evening and morning activities so as to let them contribute to self-loving transition times.

Also consider the kind of space you like to sleep in. Sleep and fantasy go hand in hand. Do you like a light, airy space? A small, cozy one? With a little ingenuity, you can customize the space around your bed to delight you. You might want to bypass the normal bedroom altogether, and create a special alcove, niche, window-seat bed, tent, or bed cabinet to accommodate just your bed and a few amenities (books, a dream journal, candles). Keep in mind the need for fresh air circulation; the more confined your bed niche, the more it will need a window or other means of ventilation.

Many people believe that it is best to sleep with one's head to the north, or, secondarily, to the east. According to *feng shui*, the ancient Chinese art of placement, there is no bad orientation for sleeping; each direction is auspicious for different purposes. Find out for yourself. Notice your past patterns of sleeping-direction: do any correspond with better sleep and wakefulness? You might try, with the aid of a compass, sleeping with your head in one direction for a week or a month, then changing to another, and so on. Keep a journal of your patterns of falling asleep, dreaming, waking, and daily life in each position. When you create a bedplace, keep in mind that you may want to change head direction from time to time, and allow for flexibility.

Sleeping areas are especially important places to keep as free as possible of air-polluting materials. In sleep our bodies and minds restore themselves, and they don't need to be fighting off invaders all night long. In addition to the building materials we examined in Chapter 11, the bed and linens themselves can contain irritants.[7] The main problems come from formaldehyde (found in permanent press sheets and pillowcases), polyester fumes (from pillows, sheets, blankets, and mattresses), polyurethane foam (mattresses and pillows), flame retardants and pesticides (mattresses), and the mold and dust mites that grow in mattresses.

FOOD PREPARATION AND EATING

We know that good nutrition is essential to health, but do we realize how much the atmosphere in which food is prepared and eaten affects us? Food prepared by a distressed cook and eaten in an atmosphere of tension can be less nourishing than food cooked with love and eaten in a warm, relaxed environment. Our hungers are both physical and psychological; preparing, eating, and sharing food can either satisfy or frustrate these hungers. One study of diet and health in low-income New York City families showed (to the researchers' surprise) that "the social atmosphere of eating did more to explain health and physical growth than the amount or nutritional content of food eaten."[8] Marilyn Diamond, co-author of *Fit for Life*, agrees:

> Where food is concerned, tension is always to be avoided. No matter how good the food might be, if it is eaten under pressure or in a tense environment, it will most often spoil in an agitated digestive tract.[9]

Obviously, the desired atmosphere of love and sharing has a lot to do with relationships and individual attitudes, but the physical environment plays a role in encouraging and expressing relax-

---

[7]Gene Bruce, "The Bedroom Goes Natural," *East West,* March, 1987, p. 57.
[8]Lamb, p. 124.
[9]Harvey and Marilyn Diamond, *Fit for Life* (New York: Warner Books, 1985), p. 117.

ation, warmth, security, and accommodation. In a physical and emotional atmosphere of caring, food preparation and eating can reconnect us with the rhythms of growth and nourishment around us and remind us of our interdependence with other forms of life.

The kitchen and eating areas are often the heart of a home and the center of shared activity in a family or among friends. The accessibility of these areas to each other and to the rest of the house sets the tone for how they are used and how people feel about them. If the kitchen and eating area are physically central to the house, without being a major thoroughfare in themselves, and have good natural lighting and views, they reinforce a sense of unity and the importance of nourishment on many levels.

The degree of separation or connectedness between cooking and eating areas is an individual matter. Many people enjoy the "country kitchen," in which one room serves as hearth, kitchen, eating area, and family room. Some cooks rebel against the open kitchen, wanting privacy and freedom from distraction and not wishing to have mealtime serenity marred by views of dirty pots and pans. Some connection is important, however, both for ease of food passage to the table and in order to avoid the disjointed feeling of meals arriving full blown from out of nowhere.

Kitchen and eating areas should be organized for pleasure and convenience—not efficiency in the sense of oversimplified sterility, but with real thought for comfort and ease. A kitchen that is poorly laid out can create more tension than love. Analyze your kitchen in terms of work areas, storage convenience, and travel distances. Make sure you have work surfaces where you need them. Store foods and equipment near where they will be used and so that they can be easily reached. Consider hanging utensils on the wall where you'll need them, and having shallow cabinets that make it easy to see and reach what you need. Strike a balance between a kitchen that is too small to be relaxing and too large to be convenient.

Also look for ways to isolate some of the standard kitchen pollution sources. An enclosed porch, adjacent to kitchen work areas and vented to the outside, can contain noisemakers like the refrigerator and the food processor as well as cooking appliances that produce heat, moisture, and/or combustion products. In fact,

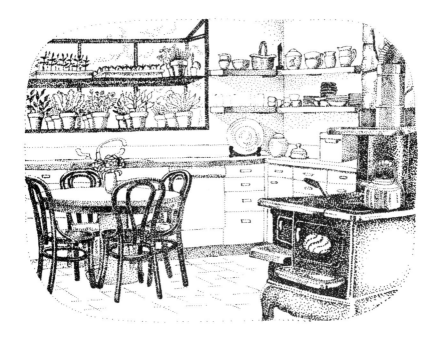

if you have the outdoor space, consider reviving the old-fashioned outdoor "summer kitchen"; it accomplishes the same indoor-pollution-abating goals, reduces the indoor cooling load in hot weather, and gets you outdoors.

Your kitchen can express your beliefs about food and nourishment. If you prefer fresh foods, you might have a garden right outside your kitchen door, or maybe an attached greenhouse or a windowsill herb garden. If food preparation is a group activity, counter space and area design can accommodate different work areas to minimize conflict. Food preparation needn't be a chore; it can be a nurturing delight.

Kitchen colors may be lively or calming, but they should never be garish or otherwise stressful, nor should they be dull. Displaying kitchen provisions on open shelves not only adds color, but increases convenience. Where shelf goods go unused for long times, glass-doored cabinets retain the visual appeal while minimizing dust problems. Ethnic cooking utensils can also be displayed, providing visual cultural links.

Eating areas are often more formal than is warranted; relaxation is more conducive to good digestion and mealtime interaction than is propriety. Architect Christopher Alexander observes:

> Some rooms invite people to eat as quickly as possible so they can go somewhere else to relax.[10]

Colors, textures, and lighting should be chosen for their warm, relaxing qualities and for the pleasant associations they evoke. A low ceiling feels cozier than a high one; the right-sized room is small enough to feel secure, but large enough to accommodate people pushing chairs back, serving food, and moving around the table without causing irritation. The best light would hang low over the table, casting enough light on the table for visibility, and giving a soft glow to the diners' faces, drawing them together.

Eating alone can also be a special experience in a pleasant atmosphere. Provide enough space, comfort, and visual interest in the surroundings to enhance a sense of self-nourishment. It's a good time to get in touch with your body and your feelings.

Recall the mealtimes of your childhood. Which aspects were pleasurable, and which not? Are you living out any of those patterns now? How could you change your eating area to minimize the unnourishing aspects and enhance the loving ones?

BATHROOMS

How you design and decorate your bathroom, and the activities you perform there, say more about your relationship with your body than does any other area. For decades, the bathroom has been the place for "unmentionables"—nudity, elimination, cleaning our private parts, and performing all kinds of reparations to keep ourselves from looking too ugly or smelling too bad—all shameful stuff to be done alone and behind closed doors, in a setting as sterile and minimal as possible.

What about a different perspective? The bathroom is a body temple, the place where we retreat ritually several times a day to reconnect with our physical nature—to experience bodily cycles, to enjoy our naked skin, to bathe languidly in warm water or

---

[10]Alexander, *A Pattern Language*, p. 844.

invigorate ourselves with a brisk shower. What if we designed bathrooms to celebrate our bodies, to allow us to do naked calisthenics, to bathe gazing at a lovely vista or a tiny bathroom garden, or to listen to soothing music? We might like a reading light and bookshelf by the tub or toilet, or room for family and friends to join us in the tub or to sit in an easy chair and converse with us.

> . . . cleaning up is only a small part of bathing; . . . bathing as a whole is a far more basic activity with therapeutic and pleasurable aspects. In bathing, we tend to ourselves, our bodies. It is one of the precious times when we are awake and absolutely naked. The relaxation of the bath puts us into sensual contact with water. It is one of the most direct and simple ways of unwinding.[11]

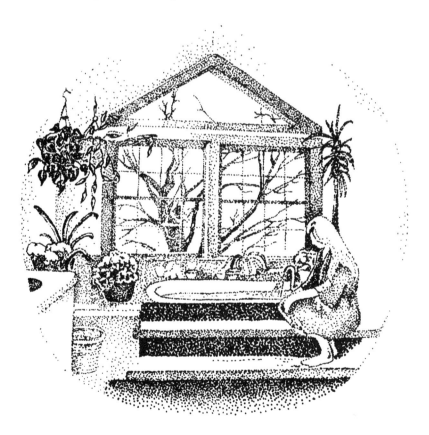

---

[11]*Ibid.*, p. 682.

In such an environment, we would want to feel reassuringly warm—radiant heat, warm floors, warm towel racks, warm surfaces. We'd want soft, warm-colored lighting to enhance our flesh tones, with brighter lights at the mirror or for reading. We'd want colors that feel warm, relaxing, and harmonious. We'd want room to move from sink to toilet to tub without bumping into hard porcelain fixtures, doors, or other people. We'd want a bathroom that says "yes" to our sensuousness, our animalness, our humanness.

Even today, as bathrooms become more colorful, more indulgent, the toilet is still an unmentionable. In larger, more communal bathrooms, it is often shut off in a separate compartment with few amenities. If toilet privacy adds to your comfort, by all means obtain it for yourself. But don't underrate the toilet experience. Many people have some of their most profound insights on the toilet. Perhaps this happens because sitting on the toilet is one of the few times in our busy days when we are absolutely where we are—fixed to the spot, in touch with our physical nature. There is a story that illustrates this phenomenon. A gentleman paid a visit to a Zen monastery, wishing to look at a famous painting there. He was told that he could not be shown the painting. In the course of his visit, he eventually had cause to visit the toilet room. As he squatted over the pit toilet, he looked up to find himself gazing at the famous painting—placed where it would be best appreciated by a person most in touch with himself.

Bathrooms are perfect places for fantasy, delight, and feeling at one with nature. Why not have a bathroom open onto a private patio garden where you can sunbathe nude? Lacking the outdoor space for that, you can turn almost any bathroom into a plant haven; vines growing along trellises above head height can hang down over the bathtub, transforming it into a grotto. Mirrors of different sizes and shapes can expand a small bathroom and allow you to appreciate your body. Displaying your favorite artwork can please your mind and focus it away from the day's toils.

A sauna might also be an appropriate adjunct to a bathroom. As used in Finland, the sauna serves many functions that are neglected in our homes. It is not only a place for deep cleansing and rejuvenation through sweating, it is also a place where family and friends gather, comfortable with their nudity, in an atmosphere of serenity. Daily rest, purification, and social bonding provide regular healing to body, mind, and spirit.

Expand your image of what a bathroom can be. Don't take anything about bathrooms for granted. Find large or small ways to satisfy your fantasies. If you are building or remodeling, consider adding space and activities to the bathroom that usually occur in other rooms, and consider separating "normal" bathroom functions into separate rooms.

One element common to all bathrooms is moisture. Our bodies and houseplants may love it, but some care must be taken to avoid mold growth and to discourage slipping in tubs and on floors. Textured (non-skid) surfaces should eliminate the latter problem. Ventilation and regular cleaning of moist nooks and crannies should discourage mold.

WORKPLACE

Throughout this book, I refer to the need for places where we can retreat, relax, and rejuvenate free of the stresses of daily life. For many of us, the greatest stressors are found where we work. If we can make our work environments less stressful, we can restore a measure of balance and wholeness to our lives, freeing up energy for fun and growth that might otherwise be spent trying to repair ourselves.

Stressors at work include noisy machinery, crowding, lack of privacy, polluted air, impersonal surroundings, inappropriate lighting, lack of contact with the outdoors, poor working postures, and a feeling of powerlessness.

Work environments cover a wide range, from factories to offices, retail stores to craft workshops. Each type of work carries its own health hazards and opportunities. Look at your present work environment from the perspective of each of the chapters in this book. Figure out where the least effort will produce the greatest benefits. If you work in a modern office building, chances are that air quality and lighting are major areas to work on, as well as the lack of arenas for self-expression in decor. In most factories,

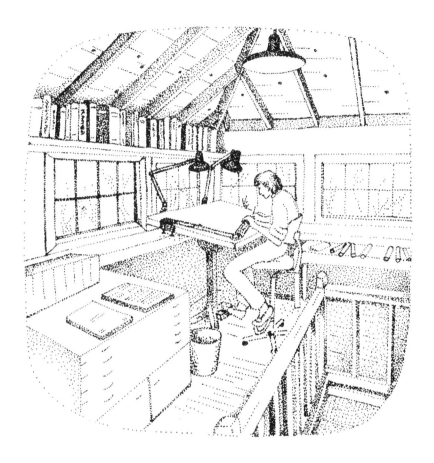

noise, air quality, and dehumanization are major health attackers. Look at the matter as a whole person who thrives with nourishment: do you want more pleasant visual surroundings, more control over your work area, livelier colors, more fresh air, greater connections with your co-workers, more flexibility in workspace layout, more privacy for creative reflection, a more restful or inspiring employee lounge, more plants?

You may have more power to affect your work environment than you realize. Some people have great freedom in outfitting their immediate work area, but make their choices based on how they will look to others rather than on whether the colors, artwork, plants, lighting, or furniture help them feel safe, integrated, creative, and happy. If you work for people who dictate every-thing from the chair you sit on to the air you breathe, you might consider educating your employers about healthy working envi-ronments. Faulty lighting, noise, poor ventilation, inappropriate temperature or humidity levels, and overcrowding cause marked drops in work efficiency. Polluted indoor air lowers productivity and increases employee absenteeism. To top it off, there is a rising tide of personal injury lawsuits as a result of poor workplace air quality, and the plaintiffs are winning. It is good business for employers to care about the healthfulness of their employees' sur-roundings.

RELAXATION

Every home and workplace needs a special place where people can retreat for relaxation. In a tense world, relaxation is one of the most effective healing tools there is. A recent study found that "twenty minutes of deep relaxation can substantially boost the body's output of immunoglobulin A—a major defense against dis-ease." The researchers concluded that "brief daily periods of re-laxation may protect individuals from illness, especially ailments of the upper respiratory tract."[12]

Dr. Herbert Benson, in *The Relaxation Response,* lists four elements necessary to effective relaxation: a quiet environment, an object to dwell upon, a passive attitude, and a comfortable position.[13] Three out of those four are directly affected by the physical environment, and the fourth (attitude) can be indirectly influenced by surroundings.

A space for relaxation should feel safe and secure. Quiet, soft light, a comfortable temperature, clean air, and calming colors (blues, greens, and lavenders) all contribute to feelings of peace-fulness and release. Soft music, plants, pleasing objects to gaze on, and a tranquil vista can heighten the experience. And, of course, the chair, mat, pillow, or whatever you sit or lie on should support you firmly, softly, and comfortably. Relaxing or meditating in the

---

[12]*Democracy at Work,* October, 1986.
[13]Donald B. Ardell, *High Level Wellness* (Emmaus: Rodale Press, 1977), p. 259.

same place regularly--especially if no other activities occur there—
will gradually build the peaceful feelings in that place, increasing
its beneficial effects over time. In a room regularly used for relaxation, merely entering the room will usually induce spontaneous
calm.

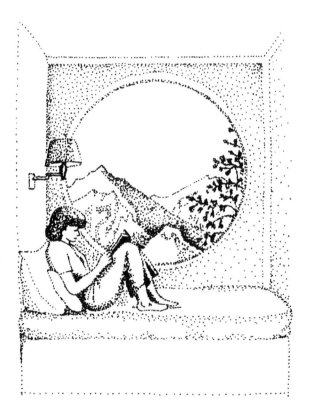

BIRTH

The environment of birth leaves a lasting impression. Its character
is crucial for both the mother and the newborn child, as well as
for others who are present. When a delivering mother is uncomfortable in the birth environment, the resulting tension translates
directly into a more difficult delivery for her and for the newborn.

Before the advent of home-like birth rooms, the typical hospital delivery room was cold, sterile, and brightly lit. Arranged for

the convenience of the hospital personnel, and dominated by emergency equipment, it spoke of a mechanized—even frightening—process. The narrow delivery table with its stirrups encouraged passivity in the mother and placed her in a physical position that was both degrading and dangerous; it diminished blood flow to the placenta, causing a drop in fetal heart rate during each uterine contraction, and prolonged labor, often producing complications.[14] Furthermore, the technological approach to childbirth traumatized both mother and child, making them less available for bonding.

Experience with more humane circumstances shows that both mothers and children tend to have fewer problems when birth occurs in a supportive environment. Sensitivity to the physical experience alone improves the situation greatly. When the mother can walk around during labor, eat, drink, visit, and give birth in whatever position she chooses, labor goes much better.[15] Attention to the physical, mental, emotional, and spiritual aspects of birth can make the experience even more positive, encouraging mother-child bonding. When the child remains with the mother immediately after birth, the bonding that comes from touching, crooning, eye contact, and smiling plays a crucial role in orienting the infant to its surroundings and establishing intimacy.[16]

The effects of environment and the mother-child relationship are observable. One study indicated that infants with more intimate postpartum contact with their mothers achieved developmental milestones significantly earlier than those who were separated by standard hospital procedures.[17] A study of French infants born by the Leboyer method—"into a warm, quiet, dimly lit delivery room, whose umbilical cords are left intact, who are given a warm bath at birth, and who are allowed virtually continuous contact with their mothers"—found the babies to appear calmer, more responsive, and more relaxed than those born

---

[14]Haire in Hastings, *Health for the Whole Person*, p. 305.

[15]Judy Goldschmidt, R.N., in Roslyn Lindheim and Shirley S. Chater, *Symposium on Environments for Humanized Health Care* (Berkeley: University of California, 1979), p. 81.

[16]Gordon in Hastings, p. 306.

[17]*Ibid.*

"among the bright lights, sharp noises, and cold surfaces of the ordinary hospital delivery room." A follow-up study found the "Leboyer children" exceptionally adroit with both hands, able to talk at an earlier age, and showing less difficulty in toilet training and in feeding themselves than the control group.[18]

CHILDREN

Children have special environmental needs. Infants with immature livers often develop jaundice if they are not exposed to full-spectrum light. Youngsters who receive the UV light so often missing indoors tend to have fewer colds, grow faster, and have better mental and physical development than those who don't. Children are also highly sensitive to temperature gradients and extremes of heat and cold. Healthy sleep can only occur when the child's body is adequately insulated but the air is not too warm.

Children tend to be more sensitive to environmental toxicity than are healthy adults. Designer Nanci Lewis of Natural Accent observes,

> You know, a mother is so excited about having a baby, she fixes the nursery up and it looks beautiful but unfortunately it's enough to make the baby sick because she's used very heavy chemical paints, chemical wallpapers, plastic furniture, or they have plastic finishes on them, she's used wall-to-wall carpet, not to mention all the synthetic stuffings in the toys and in the bumper pads . . .[19]

Children also have unique neurological needs which too frequently go unmet. According to child psychiatrist Reginald S. Lourie, the infant is born with an "unfinished" brain, and takes one-and-one-half to two years after birth to reach the level of maturity that is typical of the time of birth in other mammals. To accomplish this, the brain is growing faster in these first two years than it ever will again, reaching more than two-thirds of its adult size. Lourie says, "Appropriate environmental experience is nec-

---

[18]*Ibid.*

[19]Debra Lynn Dadd, "The Beauty of Nature in Your Home, An Interview With Nanci Lewis," *Everything Natural,* July/August, 1987, p. 17.

essary for the stimulation of the embryonic genetic mechanisms to complete their unfolding tasks."[20]

Psychologist H.P. Schaffer observed infants under seven months old who were hospitalized for one to two weeks in a typical monotonous hospital environment. After returning home, these infants continued to stare into space with blank expressions on their faces for a few hours to a couple of days.[21] Psychologist M.D. Vernon's response to these findings was:

> Thus we must conclude that normal consciousness, perception, and thought can be maintained only in a constantly changing environment. When there is no change, a state of 'sensory deprivation' occurs; the capacity of adults to concentrate deteriorates, attention fluctuates and lapses, and normal perception fades. In infants who have not developed a full understanding of their environments, the whole personality may be affected, and readjustments to a normal environment may be difficult.[22]

The development of the infant's brain is not thoroughly understood, but three basic processes have been identified which, in addition to genetic potential, determine the brain's level of function:

1. The number of connections that grow between brain cells is determined by the amount and type of stimulation available in the first years of life; the more connections formed, the greater the possibilities for flexibility, integration of functions and information, creativity, and the possibilities for choice in the individual.

2. The amount of blood flow to the different centers of function in the brain is developed in proportion to the amount of appropriate stimulation of each function.

3. Nerve networks and connections develop without an outer coating which must be formed before the nerve can be ac-

---

[20]Reginald S. Lourie, "Consideration for the Young in a City for Human Development," *Ekistics*, April, 1973, p. 221.

[21]Faber Birren, "The Significance of Light: Reactions of Mind and Emotion." *AIA Journal*, October, 1972, p. 39.

[22]*Ibid.*

tivated for use by the individual. This process is considerably influenced by environmental stimulation, with significant effects on ultimate structure and function. Deprivation can result in developmental delays and poorer functioning.[23]

By one estimate, 3% to 5% of the United States population is mentally retarded, three-fourths of which is due to inappropriate or deficient experience in the first years of life.[24]

Lourie suggests that, in the home, the infant should be near the center of activity. With a bassinet or playpen in the kitchen, the baby can make connections between the smell, taste, and looks of the food, as well as imprinting the parents' moves and activities. "He can then learn quite early how to communicate, even when to curse, such as when a pot falls and spills. Also, the attachment process can be enhanced, as well as the knowledge that mothering is available on shorter notice than when the infant is off in a bedroom."[25]

Children also need basic outdoor experiences, such as how earth feels and that plants grow. Playgrounds can allow for learning and for experiencing body movement. Environmental Psychologist Maxine Wolff says, "[Play] can help to promote personal confidence in relationships with others. It can serve to minimize the poverty of environmental information to which [children] have access by promoting exploration and manipulation through experimentation."[26] This implies that the play area contains novelty, information, complexity, and opportunity.

Biologist Rene Dubos has observed that New York's Lower East Side produced that city's richest number of creative people around the turn of the century, despite its deficiency of desirable physical qualities. He also found the small family farm to be "immensely creative." "What do the Lower East Side and the American family farm . . . have in common? Both situations not only

---

[23]Lourie, *Ibid.*

[24]*Ibid.*

[25]*Ibid.*

[26]Wolff in David Canter and Sandra Canter, *Designing for Therapeutic Environments* (Chichester: John Wiley & Sons, 1979), p. 89.

provide a wide range of experiences, but they both demand that the child act and function; that he does something and he is able to see the results, the consequences."[27]

THE ELDERLY

We all grow older, but few of us look forward to our "golden years" with glowing anticipation. Our culture has relegated the elderly to the shadows in a way that is damaging to all of us at every age. The built environment is only part of the problem, but this is a clear case of how social priorities have produced places that are hostile to an entire phase of human life.

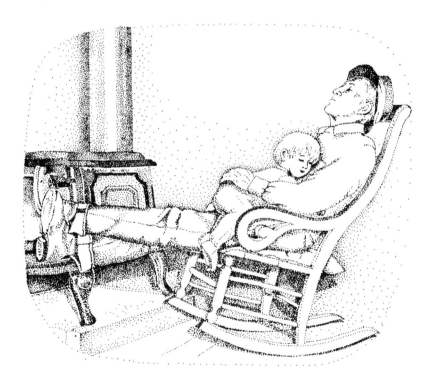

---

[27]Rene Dubos, "The Biological Basis of Urban Design," *Ekistics*, April, 1973, p. 201.

Health writer Ken Dychtwald, Ph.D., aptly describes the situation:

> Most environments seem tailored to people with a standard size and a specific range of mental and neurological abilities. Our contemporary cities are like monstrous cookie cutters shaped to exclude people who cannot function within certain limited physical parameters. Many older people . . . cannot attend public events because the transportation is inappropriate, the walkways too slippery, the rooms too dark, or the lettering on the signs too small. There are often no elevators and the bathrooms are too hazardous. . . .[A]s one ages, environments that were once comfortable and supportive become transformed into dark, slippery, crime-ridden, scarcely navigable obstacle courses. . . .
>
> [Older people] internalize the message that they do not belong in the world. Where outrage would be an appropriate and reasonable response, we too often see resignation, sickness, low self-esteem, and anomie. In time, continued interaction with these negative images and structures directly translates into frustration, tension, unhappiness, loneliness, stress, and a decreased will to live.[28]

Old age can be a time of flourishing and fulfillment in a social and physical environment that acknowledges the uniqueness of the later years of life. For most, it is a time of increased personal maturity and decreased responsibilities—a fertile combination. If we don't relegate the elderly to deadly institutions, and if we consider the full span of life when we create our homes, public buildings, and outdoor spaces, the potential vitality of the elderly can be available to enrich everyone's life.

Environments that are accommodating to the elderly can make the difference between precarious health and full functioning. Whether you are planning for your own later years or for someone else's, it's worth keeping some basic principles in mind:

Vision. Aging is often accompanied by a loss of visual acuity, narrowing of the visual field, slowed accommodation to temporal or spatial changes in illumination, sensitivity to glare, and diminished color differentiation.[29] Increased lighting levels—with caution to avoid glare—solve many "poor vision" problems; this is crucial in stairways, bathrooms, kitchens, and reading areas. Well-

---

[28]Dychtwald in Hastings, p. 365.
[29]Laszlow Aranyi and Larry L. Goldman, *Design of Long-Term Care Facilities* (New York: Van Nostrand Reinhold Company, 1980), p. 31.

designed lighting can also contribute to the overall pleasantness of the environment. Where signs are used, they should have large lettering in strong contrast to its background. Color can enliven an area and give a sense of orientation by enhancing the contrast between surfaces or when different areas or functions are color coded.

Thermal comfort. The elderly are more likely to complain of being too cold than too warm, typically requiring temperatures five degrees higher than younger people.[30] Protection from extremes of both heat and cold is also important. Humidity should be controlled to avoid respiratory illness, dehydration, and static electricity problems.

Maneuvering. Non-skid surfaces, an absence of sharp corners, abundant handrails, clear pathways, resting places on long halls or stairways, and accommodation for wheelchairs, canes, and "walkers" can minimize injuries and frustration.

Orientation. Mental confusion can be reduced if one is frequently given clues by one's surroundings as to who and where one is. Views to the outdoors provide reminders of locale, season, weather, and time of day. Each room or area can have its own colors, lighting, and textures, increasing its identifiability.

Dignity. The environment should be structured to allow a person both privacy and interaction at will. It should allow one to carry out useful and meaningful activities. And it should enable one to continue to feed, clothe, bathe, and exercise oneself for as long as possible.

DYING

"Healing" and "dying" may seem at first to be antithetical notions. But dying is part of living, and tremendous mental, emotional, and interpersonal healing can occur in the dying process— not only for the dying person, but for friends and family as well.

---

[30]*Ibid.*, p. 34.

Reintegrating death and dying with our picture of life can heal our psyches and allow us to anticipate our own death as a natural stage of life.

One of the most fearsome aspects of death is the ignorance with which our culture tends to address it. As Norman Cousins observed,

> Death is not the ultimate tragedy of life. The ultimate tragedy is depersonalization—dying in an alien and sterile area, separated from the spiritual nourishment that comes from being able to reach out to a loving hand, separated from a desire to experience the things that make life worth living, separated from hope.[31]

Yet more positive images exist. William H. Lamers, M.D., who directs an in-home hospice program, tells of a family that came to him. They feared sending an 83-year-old family member into the impersonal atmosphere of a hospital or nursing home. Dr. Lamers helped them set up a room at home where the dying woman could be cared for by family and visiting medical people. "The woman received such magnificent care at home that the day before she died, she looked up and said, 'Dying, you know, is the experience of a lifetime.'"[32]

Philosopher Alasdair McIntyre said,

> The role of the dying man is twofold. On the one hand, he has to make that reckoning with his own past life, which is required if life is to be completed satisfactorily. . . . But, at the same time, the dying man has to hand on to the next generation the tasks and possessions that have hitherto been his; he must tell them now what he will never be able to tell them again.[33]

The atmosphere for such a passage should be familiar and comfortable—home, if possible; home-like if not. Long vistas for contemplation, plants to watch grow, favorite objects nearby, the peace of solitude, and the love and touch of family and friends can aid the knitting-together process.

When dying at home is impractical, and dying in a hospital is inappropriate, the inpatient hospice can provide a homelike at-

---

[31]Norman Cousins, *Anatomy of an Illness* (New York: W.W. Norton & Company, 1979), p. 133.

[32]Lamers in Lindheim, p. 65.

[33]Jonsen in Lindheim, p. 40.

mosphere where family and friends are welcome and the dying person can live with dignity. Deborah Carey, in her book *Hospice Inpatient Environments*, observes:

> Designing the inpatient environment includes, among other things, establishing a sense of place. Typically, individual meaning is given to a place when territory is established and embellished with personal articles, people, and memories of past events. Because hospice care is short-term, it is often hard to encourage patients and family to personalize their space. When time is short, however, as for the dying, the smallest event can take on great meaning for the dying person, the family, even the caregivers.[34]

Contemplation of nature also takes on heightened meaning for the dying. Accessible gardens, operable windows, planter boxes, houseplants, and the presence of pets can provide direct experiences. Nature-related artwork, natural color schemes, and the presence of wood, stone, and water can be suggestive. As Carey notes,

> Human beings are intimately tied up with nature. The biological processes that create us ultimately kill us; part of circumstances and cycles we are just beginning to define. Humans have been examining their place upon the earth and in the spiritual realm throughout history. . . . . Physical death summons up those connections, as we struggle to understand our lives and the purpose of existence.[35]

---

[34]Deborah Allen Carey, *Hospice Inpatient Environments* (New York: Van Nostrand Reinhold Company, 1986), p. 212.

[35]*Ibid.,* p. 229.

CHAPTER 14

Design Elements

What do we know of the deeper implications
of shelter, the ecology of buildings, of the importance
of size and shape, of our relationship to ourselves
and our earth as builders?

—RIVER

Now that we've looked at some of the elements that contribute to
healthy places, and explored some ways of bringing these parts
together for specific uses, let's take another step back and look at
a larger picture. The most powerful aspects of healing environments arise from the goals and attitudes we bring to their creation. Some time-honored unifying principles can start us in the
right direction and serve as guidelines throughout the process.

Center and Boundary

One of the most basic acts in creating a place is establishing
its center and its boundaries. Without these two interdependent
features, "there is no there there." We can imagine someone about
to create a basic shelter—one that has existed, with slight variations, in cultures all over the world. The person stands in one spot
holding a long stick, and with that stick draws a circle on the
ground by turning around in place. The walls will go up where
the circle is traced, providing privacy, retaining warmth, and setting apart a space for the family. At the center of the hut will be
the fire or hearth, with a smoke hole above.

For millenia, the hearth has been the functional and symbolic center of the home. The family gathered there to stay warm, often performing tasks by the fireside while conversing and forging bonds with each other. The hearth was the center for cooking and eating, with all the attendant good smells and feelings of physical and emotional nourishment. And the flames of the fire had a magnetic, hypnotic quality, inducing revery and peacefulness in those relaxing around the fire at the day's end.

For most Americans today, cooking, eating, and physical warmth are no longer functions of the hearth fire, and yet the fireplace retains a special meaning. In many homes it is vestigial, reduced to a symbolic gesture. But its continued presence and popularity—including a recent upsurge in the use of woodstoves to heat homes—implies that we long for that traditional sense of center.

The center can take many forms. In a hot arid climate, the center may be the courtyard garden with its cooling fountain. In a spiritual community, the center might be the meditation hall. In a business place, the center could be the conference room, the employee lounge, or the coffee machine. For a contemporary family, it is often the dining area, where the family gathers daily to share food and conversation.

> In my childhood . . . we ate happily in the kitchen, surrounded by the smells—the aromatic attractions—of the meal prepared. If you ask me what home meant to me, it was that kitchen table. We played poker on it. I did my homework on it. I had coffee and discussed 'life' with my mother over it.[1]

Unfortunately, the television set has replaced both the hearth and the dining table as the center of activity in many modern homes.

The center of a home or workplace arises out of the most important shared values and activities of those who reside there. At the center, the many forces in a place come into balance. Unity is expressed and reinforced. Ideologically, for a group or an individual, the center corresponds to the heart of the group or personal identity: *Who am I/who are we; what values and activities are most meaningful to us and best express our true selves?*

---

[1]Catherine C. Crane, *Personal Places* (New York: Whitney Library of Design, 1982), p. 10.

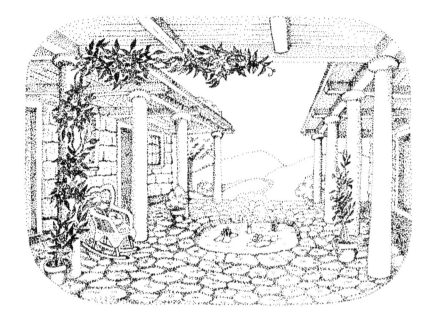

In modern Japan, where new homes are looking increasingly Western, many dwellings retain a traditionally arranged, tatami-matted room as their heart. With its simple, low furnishings, wooden beams, Shoji screens, and tokonoma (display alcove or altar), it serves as a peaceful ceremonial center for the family.

In Western culture, we often lack a strong sense of where the center is. We can discover and augment an existing center by observing our behavior and values—noticing where we gravitate, where we go to be with others or to restore ourselves, what our favorite activities are and where we go to perform them. When a natural center reveals itself, we can enhance it by making it more comfortable, by placing it in the physical center of our activities where possible, and by decorating it with colors and items that reinforce the group unity or individual sense of self.

Closely related to the question "Who am I?" (center) is the question "Who/what am I not?" This is boundary. The boundary is the functional and symbolic edge of our immediate world, the transition zone where we select who and what may enter. Boundary does not necessarily create isolation, but it is part of definition. It allows us to intensify what goes on within, whether that be keeping the space warm, enhancing group unity, focusing on work and productivity, or protecting possessions from burglars. Healthy boundaries also improve the relationship between what's inside and what's outside by encouraging connections that are mutually respectful.

Boundary may seem more obvious than center—after all, if you're making a building, you're usually putting up walls. But the important thing is to consider carefully the nature of that boundary. Do the walls we live inside represent the choices we would make consciously about what to have within and what to keep out? Have we placed those walls so that they contain our activities in supportive ways? Do these boundaries respond to the terrain, the climate, the vistas, and the life forms around them? Do we feel trapped inside the walls, or protected and nurtured?

The expressions of center and boundary in our physical environment mirror and shape our personal sense of self, from which our health and well-being derive. Knowing who we are and the difference between "self" and "other" is the basis of the creative drive and the will to live that keep us going. Having a physical center to which we return for sustenance, and boundaries within which we are safe to be who we are, help create the self-confidence and the personal power to overcome the doubts, fears, and weaknesses that invite ill health.

Orientation

Hand in hand with the question, "Who am I?" go the questions "Where am I?" and "How do I fit into the world?" In preindustrial cultures worldwide, people have oriented their lives and buildings in terms of the four directions (north, east, south, and west), the heavens, and landscape features such as a mountain or river. Cities and whole nations were divided into quadrants, often with gates opening to each of the four directions. Homes and religious structures were laid out in relation to the rising and setting of the sun. We now need that feeling of relationship with the whole as much as ever; it gives us a context, a sense of rightful participation in the universe.

Though every culture has attached different specific meanings to the four directions, the basic connotations are universal: the east is the direction of the rising sun, symbolizing beginnings, illumination, birth and rebirth, vision, and the awakening of mental powers; the south[2] is the direction of warmth, growth, activity, physicality, and climax; the west is the setting sun, and the direction of repose, reflection, completion, release, and putting things in order; the north is quiet, stillness, dark, cold, inner focus, and passivity.

The meanings of the four directions are highly practical; we want to orient our rooms and our activities to harmonize with their qualities. We work best with nature when we awaken and begin our days with east light, carry out our main activities with south light (except in hot seasons), repose at the end of the day with relaxing west light, and retreat from activity by moving into a north-facing room. This is an oversimplified picture, but it provides a basis for considering our daily cycle of activities in relation to the cycles of the sun. There is a deep satisfaction that comes from being aware of where the sun is in its path and attuning ourselves to it.

Not only may we place our rooms and activities so as to admit or exclude sunlight and locate our windows to let us see the sun and moon rise and set, but we can also create alignments that increase our contact with seasonal cycles and heavenly events. We can look to our ancestors who erected stone circles, temples, and burial chambers to serve as living calendars. In many cave temples, for example, a single opening admitted a beam of sunlight that shone directly on the altar at sunrise on a particular day of the year, marking the time for rituals appropriate to the season. Alignments of stones allowed priests to track the return of a significant star or planet to a particular spot in the sky.

In our recent past, with the use of central heating and electric lighting, caught up in high-pressure lifestyles oriented around cars, television, and indoor jobs, we've lost touch with the daily and seasonal cycles of sun, moon, and stars. Physiologically and psychologically, the effects on our functioning are probably greater than we suspect. The use of solar energy—particularly design of buildings for passive solar heating and natural cooling—is a powerful step in the direction of reconnecting us with planetary forces.

---

[2]In the southern hemisphere, the meanings of south and north would be reversed.

It can be the beginning of a new cosmic perspective.

As we explore our relationship with the motions of the stars and planets, and as we allow our buildings to express those connections, we may find levels of meaning in life that we have forgotten. Our sense of self might strengthen, our biological clocks could function more effectively, and our place in the web of life would feel more real.

In addition to the four directions, towns and buildings have often been oriented to prominent landscape features. A town laid out between two hills or along a riverbank has a sense of place that it would otherwise lack. When we have a view from our home or workplace of a distant mountain or a distinctive tree, we develop a relationship with it over time. It helps us to know where we are, and perhaps to contact a sense of time and timelessness.

Begin to explore the worlds outside your walls, looking for ways to let in more awareness of direction, cycles, and landmarks. Think about which times of day, seasons, and places have special meaning for you, and imagine ways in which you can honor those events through your environment.

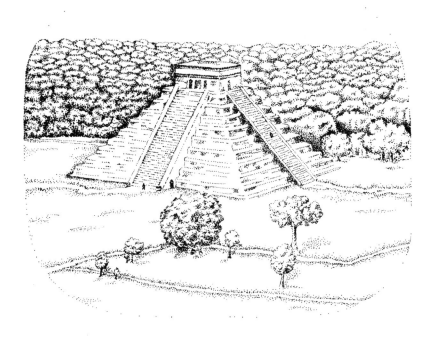

Place Energy

Can you recall an occasion when you walked into an unfamiliar room and immediately felt welcome and comfortable there? Or perhaps another time when you entered a place and felt a foreboding that you couldn't shake? Places can have an essence that goes beyond their physical characteristics. We sense that essence—which some people call "place energy"—all the time, but our awareness of it usually remains semi-conscious. Even so, we respond via our actions. By observing our behavior and that of others, we can begin to see the subtle forces at work: in most rooms, there are spots where no one lingers and areas where people gravitate; we often have a favorite chair in a special spot where we go to relax; and, as with Winnie-the-Pooh's friend Christopher Robin, there's a particular step on the staircase where it feels best to sit.

We feel the extremes most readily—a sense of peace and upliftment in Chartres Cathedral, or tension and anguish at the site of a past calamity. Through attention and practice we can learn to acknowledge the subtle but powerful currents that run through our everyday surroundings. When we recognize and work with healthful, loving energy, we can better locate and create healing places.

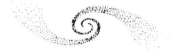

The best tool for discerning place energy is yourself: your body, emotions, instincts, and thoughts. Scan the area where you are, using not just your eyes but your whole being. Notice what spot or direction you are drawn toward. Release yourself from strictly visual/mental attraction such as "What a pretty plant; I think I'll go there" or "That looks like a comfortable chair." Look for the spot where you feel most "right"—most whole, content, and centered. When you find your spot, you will feel that you have arrived; you won't be eager to get up and move. It may take several tries before you come to the spot; it may even be a while before you recognize that "right" feeling when it happens. But as you practice, you'll naturally begin to seek out the most comfortable

spot for you wherever you are. This is a very personal exercise; different people feel good in different places. And you will find that there are different "right" spots for different purposes. In my house, for instance, there is a place that feels right for meditation, another for writing, another for socializing, and so on. It took me a while to catch on that the place where I first put my desk wasn't working out, and that it really felt best as a meditation spot, but once I sorted it out, the increased sense of harmony was a great relief.

Many factors go into creating the energy of a place. Orientation, light, color, sound, symbol, materials, form, climate, vista, and electromagnetism combine to make each spot unique. The activities that occur and the feelings people have in a place add another layer, leaving echoes of happiness or misery in the walls. The landscape and the elements have their own inherent feelings that set the tone for any activity or construction.

Ancient cultures have traditionally acknowledged the special qualities of certain places. Some locations were believed to aid in healing or to heighten spiritual awareness; others were thought to be areas of illness and bad fortune. Temples were usually situated in spots that had especially powerful spiritual energy; such considerations governed the siting of structures as diverse as British stone circles, Egyptian pyramids, Mayan and Incan temples, American Indian stone medicine wheels, the Palaces of China, and the Gothic cathedrals of Europe.

Various pre-industrial cultures developed their own science and art of perceiving the energies and rhythms of the earth and cosmos, and of prescribing the layout of habitations to harmonize human activity with natural patterns. These practices are known as "geomancy," which means "divining the earth spirit." "Geomancy seeks the harmonious placement of cities, buildings, and human activities, so that the vitality of the earth's life force . . . is maintained."[3] The Chinese evolved a detailed form of geomancy known as "feng shui," meaning "wind and water." Feng shui de-

---

[3]Richard feather Anderson, "Divining the Spirit of Place." *Yoga Journal*, September/October, 1986, p. 27.

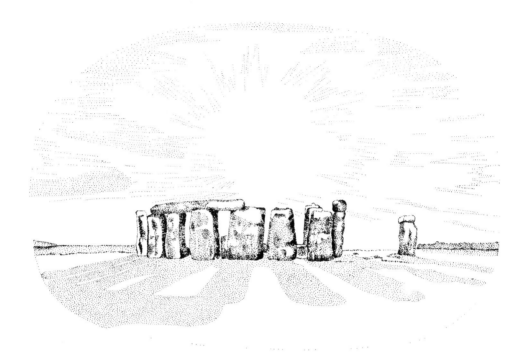

veloped from the observation that people's health and fortunes were affected by their surroundings—where their buildings were located in the landscape, and how their homes and workplaces were laid out.

> The application of feng shui to building location and design was based on a belief that at every place there are special topographical features, either natural or artificial, which indicate or modify the cosmic energies present there. The forms and arrangements of hills, the nature and directions of watercourses, the heights and forms of buildings, the location of forests, roads, and bridges are all important factors.[4]

Although feng shui masters are known to use special compasses and other divining tools, the abiding principle of feng shui is awareness of the flow of "ch'i," or "life force." To the Chinese, ch'i links substance and spirit.[5]

---

[4]Tom Bender, *Environmental Design Primer* (Salem, Oregon: published by the author, 1973, p. 180.

[5]Sarah Rossbach, *Feng Shui: The Chinese Art of Placement* (New York: E. P. Dutton, Inc., 1983), p. 23.

> Ch'i is everywhere, in people as in things; it is as much the magnetism
> that moves the geomancer's compass needle, as the beauty of a scene
> that commands an artist's awe.[6]

The goal of the feng shui master is to tap the earth's ch'i, finding
a place for habitation where the ch'i flows smoothly and the principles of yin (passive) and yang (active) are in balance. Where such
a site is not available, feng shui provides means of altering or
responding to imbalances, bringing the environment into harmony.

These practices are neither entirely mystical nor entirely ex-
plicable. Viewed from today's perspective, much of the advice of
a feng shui master is good common sense: locate your house part
way up a south-facing slope overlooking water that moves neither
too quickly nor too slowly. The south orientation invites the sun's
warmth; the slope behind the house protects it from cold winds;
the water will bring cooling summer breezes, while being neither
stagnant nor menacing. But other aspects of feng shui are not as
tangible; in directing good ch'i to a person, or diverting harmful
ch'i, the master often deals with unseen forces in symbolic or
ritualized ways. It is said that the modern feng shui practitioner
can, with the appropriate placement of a mirror or relocation of
a bed, change a family's health and finances from struggling to
thriving.

How are we to apply such notions to our lives? The first step
is to gradually increase our awareness of what around us feels
beneficial or detrimental. As one feng shui expert wrote, "If a
geomancer can recognize ch'i, that is all there is to feng shui."[7]
The history of feng shui contains episodes during which its principles were interpreted as fixed rules and its spirit lost.[8] But intuition has always been the heart of feng shui, and its use will more
consistently produce balance and harmony than will any rigid
application of principles.

Once we learn to follow our intuitions, we can locate activity
areas to best advantage, placing a desk where mental activity is

---

[6]Andrew L. March, "The Winds, the Waters and the Living *Qi*," *Parabola*, Vol. III,
Issue 1, 1978, p. 29.

[7]Rossbach, p. 21.

[8]Holborn, *The Ocean in the Sand*, p. 20.

enhanced and a meditation area where spiritual focus is best attained.

In feng shui, it is believed that the ch'i inside a house or workplace must be balanced; if it is not, no amount of balance in the outside surroundings will save the inhabitants from stress, irritability, poor health, and unhappiness. In the home, the location and design of two areas is seen as most important: the master bedroom, where most adults spend at least a third of their lives; and the kitchen, where food is prepared "influencing health and, indirectly, wealth."[9]

> Interiors with good feng shui nourish the residents' ch'i, so they will both thrive in the outside world and handle hostile circumstances ranging from gun-point robberies to cutting tongues.[10]

While becoming aware of place energy and learning to work with it can be an intensely personal experience, it can simultaneously unite us with the greater whole. We cannot long attend to healthful flows without acknowledging that all of life and the earth are related via this life force. Working with place energy is the ultimate example of the double meaning of "healing environments;" the practice of feng shui aims not only to provide auspicious locations for human settlements, but largely to "maintain the ch'i, or life force, of the living earth."[11] That life force creates and is nourished by the sun, moon, earth, winds, waters, seasons, and life forms. The character of our lives and cultures corresponds directly to our attunement with or alienation from these forces. Our thoughts and actions either honor or ignore this spirit that flows through and around us.

Form

The shape of a room or a building may also influence how you feel there. Naturalist May Theilgaard Watts observed that the square—which, with its cousin the rectangle, forms the basis of nearly all modern buildings—rarely appears in living things. When

---

[9]Rossbach, p. 78.
[10]*Ibid.*, p. 103.
[11]Anderson, p. 56.

it does, she says, it is always softened by flowing contours. The spiral, the circle, the five-pointed star, and the triangle, however, appear over and over.[12] Some people believe that rectangular enclosures produce eddies of stagnant energy in their corners.[13] By contrast, dwellers in yurts and tipis often report feeling greater

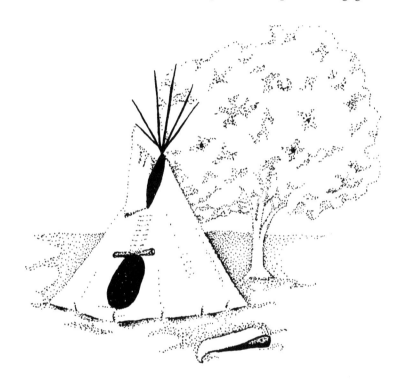

wholeness and continuity—a "better-rounded energy" than they did in rectilinear structures. Native American Black Elk observed that "the Power of the World always works in circles;" that "there can be no power in a square."

> Our teepees were round like the nests of birds, and these were always set in a circle, the nation's hoop, a nest of many nests, where the Great Spirit meant for us to hatch our children.

---

[12]May Theilgaard Watts, *Reading the Landscape* (New York: The MacMillan Company, 1957), p. 192.

[13]Anderson, p. 56.

But the Wasichus [white men] have put us in these square boxes. Our power is gone and we are dying, for the power is not in us any more.[14]

Other cultures have found power in juxtaposing the square and the circle, often by placing a hemispherical dome over a rectilinear building. The dome of heaven rests above the base of the earth, balancing masculine and feminine energies, and integrating human life, earth, and heaven.

Rectilinear buildings constructed according to the ratio 1:1.618 are said to produce a sense of peace and integration by their harmonious proportions. This is the "golden section" or "divine proportion" found often in nature and used in the design of

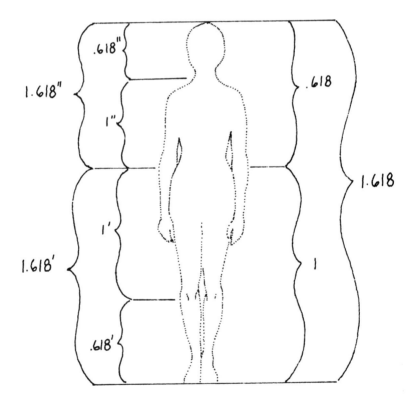

[14]John G. Neihardt, *Black Elk Speaks* (New York: Washington Square Books, 1959), p. 164.

early European cathedrals, Egyptian pyramids, Greek temples, and numerous modern buildings.

Pyramids, octagons, cones, domes, and divinely proportioned boxes have all been credited with the powers to produce beneficial effects in people. Some may be best used at special healing and spiritual spots where people come to soak up intensified, focused energy. Others may be more balanced, appropriate to harmonizing daily life. At this time, in this culture, we are exploring many forms and feelings, sometimes borrowing from other cultures, sometimes experimenting with free-form or geodesic structures.

Architect Charles Harker, of the Tao Design Group in Austin, Texas, studied organic growth processes to create a "habitable sculpture." ". . . many persons expressed feelings of 'harmony' and 'unity' while in proximity to this flowing, organic form. Others felt a 'closeness to nature.' . . . [E]motional qualities of form . . . might be developed as a means to re-establishing the psychological ties which are necessary to a healthy, symbiotic relationship of man to the natural environment."[15]

Begin to notice how you feel in spaces of various shapes and proportions. Play with changing the rooms where you live. If you find corners unpleasant, you might hang fabric to hide them, build triangular cabinets to blunt them, or even put up wire mesh and plaster to turn them into curves. If you are creating a new structure, explore a range of possibilities before you settle on the forms that feel right for your life and your site.

Balance

Balance is not symmetry. It is not static; it is flow in harmony. Things are always in motion, but balance must be maintained for life to thrive. Our organisms require balanced input and outflow. In our world, we need balance between earth and sky, activity and rest, order and chaos, dark and light, social and private, inner and outer, familiarity and change, yin and yang.

Look at your present surroundings in terms of balance. Does your environment offer you opportunities for work and for rest? For external focus and internal direction? To gather with others

---

[15]Charles Harker, "Psychosynergetic Space," mimeographed, 1975, p. 2.

and to be alone? Our senses need variety and change; overstimulation and understimulation can both be harmful.

In applying the insights gained through this book, the overriding principle is to do so in a balanced way. Although we want connections with the outdoors, we also want the protection of our structures. While sunlight is healthy, too much of it will burn our skin, overheat our buildings, and create glare. Though we want peace and quiet, enduring silence can be deadly.

Balance applies to every level of environmental change. If you are planning to remodel a cherished old building, you will want to strike a balance between preserving its existing charm and altering it to meet your new needs. If you are considering restructuring your working or living place for greater efficiency and organization, you might want to reserve an area for junk and disarray.

Balance can affect our physical health, as when we seek appropriate thermal, sonic, and luminous inputs. But esthetic and "sensed" balance can also influence our well-being by putting our minds at ease.

Love

Love is the magic ingredient in any environment. Loving the place where you are, loving yourself, and sharing love with others all build up the good feelings in a place, making them available to all who enter. The loving energy that goes into creating an environment—from shaping its overall form to handcarving a cabinet door handle—will be evident for as long as the building stands.

Love means taking the care to notice what really pleases you and the people around you, and providing those things for yourselves, to serve you and bring you joy every day. It means not just doing the standard thing or the fashionable thing, but exploring yourself and your world to create wonderful things, the things you desire most in your true self, the things that reflect back to you who you really love being.

If you put a little extra energy into special, deeply satisfying things—and don't waste your energy on things you have no need for—you can create a uniquely nourishing environment. This might mean creating a cozy nook for curling up and reading a book, an indoor jungle where you are lost in plants, a special cabinet to display artifacts or memorabilia that give you a sense of roots, a window seat for watching the world outside, or anything you can conjure up in your mind.

To stir your imagination, think back to places where you've been that warmed your heart. What qualities and features did each place have? Can you translate any of these into your present surroundings? Can you introduce something—perhaps as simple as a photograph or an object—that will remind you of that place and induce in you its peace and happiness?

Think about the things you most enjoy doing—hobbies, entertainment, reading, relaxing—and imagine ways that your environment can support those activities. It's much easier to fully enjoy yourself and whatever you are doing when the place in which you do it is accommodating.

Love within us and in our surroundings is the perfect antidote to stress, conflict, and alienation. It heals our body and our soul. It flows from us and back to us. It unites us with the universe.

· CHAPTER · 15 ·

Healing Centers

. . . a hospital is no place for a person who is seriously ill.
—NORMAN COUSINS

The focus of this book has been on making wherever you are a healing place—on letting your life, your home, and your workplace be sources of vitality and affirmation. This is a conscious attempt to counteract the possibility of making wonderful healing places for the unwell while neglecting our daily environments. If all our love and wisdom about creating healing environments is focused on recovery from or treatment for illness, we create rewards for illness. We may perpetuate a tendency for people to become ill as a way of satisfying basic desires for loving attention, relaxation, and an escape from dehumanizing forces in their daily lives.

In any society, however, there are times when we need the care of a healer, when we need activities and education to improve our well-being, when we need a place to cleanse our bodies of environmental pollutants, or when we need a mental break from our usual surroundings. Healers—whether physicians, massage therapists, psychic healers, psychologists, nutritional advisors, herbalists, chiropractors, acupuncturists, or any of a number of other practitioners—have an important role in our lives, and the environments in which they work with clients and take care of themselves can augment or detract from the effectiveness of their treatments.

A healing center can be anything from a single room where a healer receives clients, to an extensive complex where many healers work. It can be a drop-in office or a residential center or both. It can be in the city or in the country. Each healer or group of healers will strive for a different type of setting, depending on the nature of their work and of their clientele. But one basic tenet should underlie their planning: that the environment should not conflict with the goal of healing, and that every opportunity should be explored for creating an environment that plays an active, positive role in the healing process. In a place of healing, the place itself must heal.

The most healing things are those that restore wholeness and connectedness. To enter a building that ignores the basis of healing, go down a hall, and wait in a room where a specialist eventually examines you and gives you something to make you feel better is like trying to paddle upstream in a flood. You have already received and processed countless messages about your powerlessness and separateness.

Most hospitals are good examples of how not to create healing environments. They seem to say, "The power here resides with the institution; the important people are the doctors; you represent an illness, and we have tests, drugs, and machinery to control it." Visually, most hospital rooms are sterile and monotonous, laid out for the convenience of the staff. Contact with the outdoors, sunshine, and growing things is rare. The air often carries toxic cleaning solutions and even germs and bacteria inadvertently ducted in from labs and other wards. Sleep is interrupted by noises or by unexpected jabs from a needle or a thermometer. In many circumstances, the patient's auditory world is disturbed by sounds from other beds and distorted by bedside machinery that whirs, bleeps, or clicks; muffled whispers and footsteps prevail, but little useful information is directed to the patient. Patients rarely have control over either their environment or their treatment.

The hospital is a place where people go after their health has reached an alarming state; it rarely plays a positive role in maintaining a person's health. Many recent attempts to improve the hospital environment have been cosmetic, not addressing the basic premises of the hospital concept.

> When staff and patients have found the hospital environment oppressive and inhumane, floors have been carpeted, walls painted bright colors, supergraphics added, but nothing fundamentally changed. While such

cosmetic improvements are important, they fail to address problems of scale or to facilitate personalized patient care.[1]

Physician Leonard Duhl points out that rather than ask, for example, how to design a better coronary care unit, we should be asking ourselves whether "the unit itself, which puts people into a very dependent situation and disconnects people from the broader community environment, may be perpetuating the potential for coronaries."[2]

Some people propose that the best centers for health promotion are the ones most integrated with the community, decentralized, familiar or homey, and encouraging healthful activities. An excellent example of this was the Peckham Health Center in England:

> The Peckham Center was a club, run by two doctors, focused on a swimming pool, a dance floor, and a cafe. In addition, there were doctor's offices, and it was understood that families—never individuals— would receive periodic check-ups as part of their activities around the swimming and dancing. Under these conditions, people used the center regularly, during the day and at night. The question of their health became fused with the ordinary life of the community, and this set the stage for a most extraordinary kind of health care.[3]

Christopher Alexander's *A Pattern Language* proposes that health centers be "as close as possible to people's everyday activities" and "able to encourage people in daily practices that lead to health"; each center should have "some functions that fuse with the ordinary course of local work and recreation: swimming pool, workshops, sauna, gym, vegetable garden, greenhouse . . . knit together loosely with other parts of the town," not forced into a continuous "health park."[4] Many types of residential care facilities—for the elderly, the physically disabled, or the mentally impaired—are more effective when they function as a part of their community; residents' health benefits from the stimulation and from the ability to pursue normal activities outside the care facility.

---

[1]Lindheim, *Symposium on Environments for Humanized Health Care*, p. 25.

[2]Leonard J. Duhl, M.D., *Making Whole* (manuscript, University of California, 1980), p. 266.

[3]Alexander, p. 254.

[4]*Ibid.*, p. 252-5.

At the same time, there is a need for healing centers that serve as retreats. Sometimes we need to get away from familiar surroundings for a fresh perspective or to escape city congestion, noise, and pollution. At a rural healing center, we can bathe in sunlight, fresh air, peaceful sounds, and open vistas. Such healing centers can function as care facilities for people with illnesses, as rejuvenation retreats for those who need occasional reattunement, and as conference centers for intensive health education.

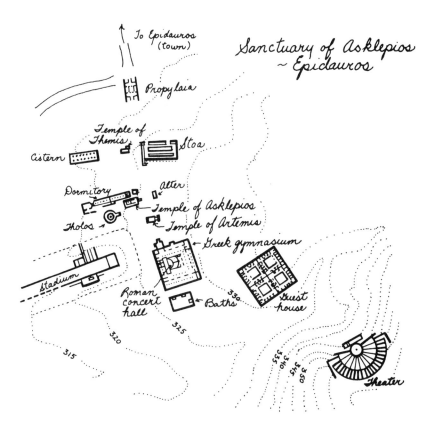

Ancient Greeks created a network of rural healing temples called "aesculapia" that can still be models for us today. There were 300 to 400 aesculapia in active use from the end of the sixth century BC to the end of the fifth century AD. These temples were dedicated to Aesculapius, the god of healing. Devotees journeyed to the temples in times of illness or crisis, or when in need of spiritual guidance, staying for days or weeks at a time. Temples were often nestled in a cypress grove near the ocean, with buildings oriented toward the sun and the fresh prevailing breezes, in harmony with their natural setting. The building complex encouraged a wide range of activities, with its library, gardens, baths, temples, open altars, sleeping rooms, gymnasium, theater, and stadium. Upon entering the temple, patients shed their clothes, bathed in the purifying water of the fountains, and donned simple robes. They fasted or ate cleansing foods, engaged in athletics or dancing, received teachings from the priests, and partook of the

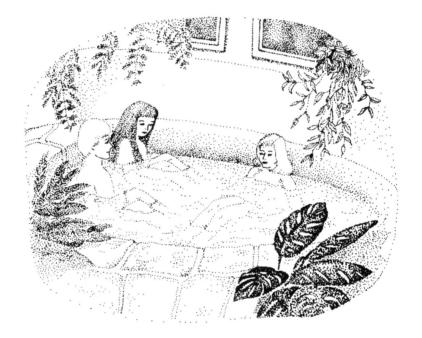

abundant art, music, and theater events—all activities designed to restore the body's rhythms and reachieve harmony of mind and body.

But the pivotal concern at the aesculapia was the dream state; diet, exercise, and ritual were all geared toward "incubating" the healing dream sought by the devotee. After several days' stay at the temple, a person performed certain sacrifices and rituals, and then entered the sacred dormitory to sleep. Spontaneous healing often occurred in the dream. In other cases the dream contained a message or guidance in the proper course for healing. Priests were available to help translate dreams into prescriptions. The temple walls were lined with inscriptions describing the cures obtained through these dreams.

Our nearest contemporary equivalent to the aesculapia might be the health spas. The Golden Door in Escondido, California is said to be one of the best; it exemplifies several principles that are worthy of emulation. The building complex is modeled on the old inns of Japan; the architecture, color scheme, plantings, and water gardens all reinforce feelings of tranquility and delight. Upon entry, guests cross a Japanese footbridge and exchange street shoes for slippers—an important transition ritual to reinforce the specialness of the retreat. During their week's stay, guests are expected to devote their time and energy to their "own life force and to emerge . . . renewed and recharged."[5] Activities involve a range of indoor and outdoor exercise, dance, massage, relaxation, herbal wraps, and meditation. "The goal is to obtain balance—a balance between exterior and interior, between activity and rest, between work and play. The result is serenity and oneness with nature—a balanced life."[6]

Spas such as the Golden Door can function well as preventive health care retreats. But for those with more serious illnesses to cure, Dr. Dorothy Waddell describes an existing "alternative" care unit in a country hospital clinic. Practitioners there believe that patients must take part in their own healing in order to produce a lasting therapeutic change. The individual is encouraged to gain a sense of control, including awareness of what is happening in his or her body and how to respond to it.

> The spaces in our unit are designed to facilitate the [mobilization of active will] and are intended to make people feel comfortable, not threatened. People comment frequently on how good they feel being there. We have space in the old hospital—funky but very nice. It includes a fireplace paved with earth-colored tiles in the seminar room, carpets on the floors, windows that open wide, old-fashioned floor-to-ceiling cupboards in the exam rooms. . . . We have a large space for seminars in which people may sit on the carpeted floor, lie, recline, twist, bend

---

[5]Emily Wilkens, *Secrets From the Super Spas* (New York: Grosset & Dunlap, 1976), p. 104.

[6]*Ibid.*, p. 108.

into yoga postures, perform Feldenkrais movements, or engage in any of a variety of maneuvers in which awareness comes through breathing, stretching, and moving. This room also provides an environment in which there is a sense of complete personal security so that, with eyes closed, people may move safely into the very special and very personal inner space of complete relaxation.[7]

In this care unit, many healing techniques are applied: relaxation, biofeedback, imagination and visualization, massage, acupuncture, acupressure, and movement training, including Feldenkrais and Alexander techniques. In the reception area, people may read from a collection of books ranging from the technical to the inspirational, or purchase relaxation tapes and paperback books.

The creators of a new healing center need first to agree on some basic principles. The best healing environments reflect an awareness of the multi-faceted humanity of individuals, whether clients or staff. Opportunities to experience oneself in a variety of contexts, to explore connections with other people and the greater pulse of life, and to gain a feeling of capability in relation to one's health will improve the outlook of everyone at the center. A client needs a sense of control and participation, a means of gaining information to help make sense of what is going on inside. If such principles are explored and agreed upon at the outset, they can be effective guides in making the specific choices that will follow.

First of all, a client needs to feel welcome. When coming to a healing center, a client is entering a foreign environment, often with fears; the transition can be eased by creating an entry area that reassures and comforts the client and creates a sense of belonging.

One way a healing center can reflect the whole person is to provide variety and flexibility. Especially in a residential center or one to which people come frequently, clients will thrive with opportunities for both privacy and interaction, relaxation and physical activity, individual attention and group experiences, security and challenge. This implies having a range of spaces, from private rooms for consultation, meditation, or sleep, to larger spaces for classes, group exercise, or sharing meals.

Opportunities for useful occupation will also increase a

---

[7]Lindheim, p. 181.

client's sense of worth, overcoming the patient passivity common in most medical clinics and hospitals. Gardening is a perfect outlet. Whether in urban or rural centers, space can usually be found for decorative or edible plants. Tending to plants and watching them grow is one of the most therapeutic activities there is. Working in a vegetable garden—whether a rooftop city garden or a country one—provides physical exercise in the sunshine and re-forges our connection with natural growth cycles and the sources of our nourishment. (See Chapters 12 and 13).

Each chapter in this book can be examined and integrated in the creation of a healing center. The place should have human scale, appear accessible, and avoid being imposing, monolithic, or confusingly complicated; it can empower the client. The thermal environment can be varied and may augment feelings of connection with nature and awareness of internal and external cycles. Natural lighting should be abundant, and artificial lighting kind and gentle; where visual tasks are performed, lighting should not strain the eyes. Colors are important and will differ from area to area: for reassurance and a sense of solidness use earthy colors; for relaxation or meditation use tints of blues, greens, and lavenders; for activity and vitalization, accents of bright, warm reds, oranges, and yellows are appropriate. Sounds should be gentle and harmonious. The air should be as free of toxic substances and allergens as possible; building materials, finishes, and furnishings should be chosen for both esthetic appeal and lack of inherent pollutants. And from location to overall form to choice of paints, every choice should be made in the context of the whole.

· CHAPTER · 16 ·

Taking Action

The creative person loves the challenge
of making chaos into form.
—ROLLO MAY

There you sit, having digested fifteen chapters of information about healing environments. You've come to perceive your surroundings in different ways, and you've learned new things about yourself. Your awareness and appreciation of the worlds within and around you have deepened and become more subtle; your priorities may even have changed. You may be excited, encouraged, and ready to forge ahead, or you may feel overwhelmed and confused, wondering where to go from here.

Perhaps you've noticed that if you wanted to apply every suggestion in this book literally, you'd be doing a lot of contradictory things. Exhaust fans provide helpful ventilation, but they can be noisy; houseplants might heal your psyche, but they tend to grow mold on their soil; painting a room blue may calm you, but the paint itself could poison you. How are you to pick a path through all the choices? By clarifying the priorities that arise from your unique needs and circumstances.

This is a good time to relax and take stock of the insights and knowledge you've gained as you read this book and to integrate them with your present situation. Wherever you are, there are things you can do to heal your environment and yourself. Whether you own or rent your home, whether you work in a highrise or a garage, whether your health is poor or excellent, whether you have a little money or a lot, you can devise a course of action appropriate for you.

You needn't fragment yourself by attempting to act on each aspect of the environment separately. Elegant solutions solve multiple problems with one action. As visionary architect Paolo Soleri once said, "I never do a thing for one reason only." For example, passive solar heating can provide healthy warmth, natural light, and contact with the sun's cycles, while not adding to the existing burdens of air pollution and fossil fuel consumption. Building with healthful techniques and materials reduces the level of toxic substances in the air, increases the life and value of a building, and can evoke a sense of satisfaction and timelessness. Appropriate use of indoor plants can enliven the visual environment, clean and humidify the air, and provide a therapeutic activity that reminds us of the wonder of life.

You don't have to take on everything at once. In fact, except in cases of major hazards, gradual changes can be the most appropriate; you avoid the trauma of having everything around you suddenly change, and you allow yourself to observe your responses to each alteration, acquiring feedback for your next step.

TAKING INVENTORY

I emphasize awareness throughout this book because it is your most valuable tool in selecting among your options. Familiarity with your resources, your health needs, your personal tastes, and your inner passions will clarify your priorities. Knowing what is most important to you serves as a guide in deciding what to do first and in facing the trade-offs that inevitably accompany building or decorating. Acting from self-awareness makes the whole process personally meaningful and produces an environment that communicates deeply to all who enter it.

Take as thorough an inventory as you can of yourself and your circumstances. I suggest using the following categories to begin with, but feel free to add anything that appeals to you.

1. *Personal health.* This includes your general health patterns, any environmental sensitivities you are aware of, recollections of places where you have felt best, and features you want for health improvement (e.g., more sunlight, less noise, no carpet).

2. *Present environment(s)*. Survey the places where you spend (or plan to spend) most of your time. You can look at them in terms of each chapter in this book, using the awareness exercises to evaluate symbolism, lighting, colors, and so on. You can rate each feature in terms of its healthfulness or harmfulness. This might also be a good time to perform tests for levels of radon, formaldehyde, and other indoor pollutants. Don't let this step discourage you; most buildings were not designed for health. Appreciate the beneficial features you find, and take hope from your growing wisdom about how to heal places.

3. *Available resources*. You will probably be adding to this category continually; we usually don't realize how much help we can call on. Resources include not only your financial and property assets, but also sources of information (books, periodicals, support groups, product manufacturers), friends who can help, things you own that could be put to use, skills you have, and so on.

4. *Other people*. These are the people with whom you share your environment. You may be evaluating a home where you live with family or friends, a workplace where you cooperate with co-workers, or a structure such as a school, health center, or retail store that will welcome many people. Take into account your relationships with these people and how the place can best enhance those. When possible, learn about their health needs and personal preferences, and explore how, together, you can satisfy these harmoniously.

5. *Self-awareness*. You can start with the awareness exercises in Chapter 5. Add other insights you've had as you read this book, as well as your goals, dreams, and lifestyle. List activities you enjoy, states of mind you like to achieve, and fantasies you have about your ideal environment.

This inventory is particularly useful for identifying which measures will have the greatest impact. You want to take actions that achieve the greatest results for the least effort. If your home contains a debilitating source of indoor air pollution, don't waste your energy changing the colors of the walls first. If you feel a deep need for soothing music, put your initial efforts there; then you'll feel more ready to determine the next step. When you know what's of primary importance to you, you can save a lot of effort by tackling those things first and handling secondary matters in time. And, again, priorities differ for each combination of person and place.

WHERE YOU ARE NOW

Healing a Place You Don't Own

You may feel fairly powerless if you live or work in "somebody else's place." If that feeling is sufficiently overwhelming, your first priority might be to get out. But if you're reasonably content where you are, you have a number of options for making healthy changes.

Don't underrate the simplest changes available to you. You can transform a place by changing its colors, revamping the lighting, and introducing plants. If repainting is discouraged, you can use wall hangings, colored lights, and furnishings to improve the color environment.

If toxic substances or allergens are a problem, explore with the owner, boss, or homeowner's association the possibility of sealing off the sources. If the heating system is harmful to you, try to cut yourself off from it and substitute your own heater.

If the sunlight comes into your environment in ways that run counter to your lifestyle, consider using the rooms in unconventional ways. If you want a greater sense of connection to the outdoors; try reorienting furniture for better views, placing mirrors to expand awareness of a vista, or putting planter boxes in windows for pleasant, filtered views.

If you live in a multi-unit building or share a workplace with others, you may need to involve others—including the building's owner—in your efforts. If you adopt a cooperative attitude and provide people with information, you can work together for solutions to improve conditions for everyone.

If You Own the Building

When you own your home, workplace, or other structure, you have more options available for changing your environment. Your limitations become those of the existing structure, its location, and your available time, money, and energy. You can tear out harmful materials, change the heating system, add or subtract space, put in new windows, and add a greenhouse, deck, or garden. And, of course, you can do all the things a non-owner can do as well. The design and construction process can be as minimal or as comprehensive as you want to make it.

Creating a New Building

Starting from the ground up gives you the greatest freedom to shape your environment and calls on all of your resources to meet the challenges. In this case, creating a healing environment starts from the moment you set out your priorities and continues through the process of site selection (see Chapters 10 and 11), design, building, and inhabiting.

Once you select a site, the ideal is to spend at least a year getting to know your piece of land before you begin to design a building. If you can camp on it, do so. If not, spend as much time there as you can at different times of day and in different seasons. Become familiar with the path of the sun and moon, the directions of the wind, the vegetation, the soil, and the animals that live or pass through there. Notice where your favorite spots are, and how the site relates to the rest of the world via vistas, sounds, and smells.

When you are ready to plan your building, you may discover that design freedom has both exhilarating and frustrating aspects. On one hand, you can be highly responsive to both your own desires and the special qualities of your locale; on the other hand, the range of choices can be overwhelming. Take your time. Avail yourself of educational resources, professional advice, and the wisdom of friends who've been through it already.

DESIGN

Whether you're redecorating a room or constructing a building, the design phase is where all the concepts come together. Chapters 13 and 14 provide some background about the aims of design for healing. Your inventory provides you with your own criteria. But the process remains of tying it all together and making it sing.

Most people begin to design by drawing walls. If walls are the most important thing to you, that's fine. But you are also free to start with more basic elements. Look at what is meaningful to you about your life, independent of the walls and the limitations you're accustomed to. Recall the experiences and qualities you find most fulfilling. Fantasize sequences of activities and spaces for each of the activities that will occur in this building. Look over your inventory and your awareness exercises and let your mind roam.

You might want to make a painting, poem, or diagram that expresses the essence of the place you want to create. It can serve as a touchstone as you continue to make your ideas more concrete.

You may decide to carry out the design process on your own, or you might want to get help from an architect. In the former case, you will find many books available about construction, design, and drawing that will fill in where you lack knowledge (see Resources p. 126). In the latter case, a good architect can apply years of experience to interpreting your wishes into drawings from which you can build. But in either case, remember that most people don't think in terms of designing and building for health and soul satisfaction. Keep your mind open, and don't make hasty decisions out of fear. Interview potential architects or consultants, tell them what you're up to, and don't work with anyone you don't feel comfortable with.

CONSTRUCTION

Some people view construction as dirty work and want as little to do with it as possible. Some see it as their main opportunity to shape their own environment, and throw themselves into it. Do whatever feels good to you, but however you handle it, embrace the role of the construction phase in the healthfulness of the whole project.

If you hire others to do all or part of the work, select your builders carefully. As with architects, most builders are unaccustomed to thinking in terms of health and well-being as compo-

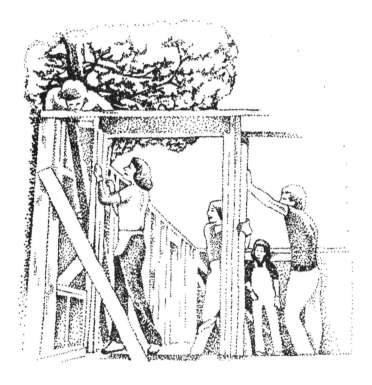

nents of a structure. If you can locate a good builder with experience in low-toxic construction, you're well ahead. But if you can't (and they're rare), look for a builder who is open to your needs and to learning new things. If you have environmental sensitivities, you may need to work closely with your builders to see that they don't unknowingly use standard materials that are harmful to you.

Choose people you can respect, and establish an atmosphere of trust. Your builders are human beings who have a role in creating a special place. Select them carefully, then work with them, not against them.

The spirit in which a building is constructed can have a powerful effect on both the process and the product. This notion is alien to most contemporary white Americans who typically pay strangers to build their structures in an atmosphere of competition, swearing, beer-drinking, loud rock 'n' roll, and louder power tools. But many traditional cultures regard the creation of a place as a sacred act. California's Pomo Indians had rules of conduct to ensure the sanctity of their building endeavors. During the construction period, people involved in a project, "must not hate another person, use vile language, take drugs, be possessed with bad thoughts or gossip, and must possess love in their hearts."[1] Others have suggested that playing beautiful music at a construction site can induce harmony in the work crew and in the building itself.

Some people are reviving the time-honored practice of bringing friends and community members into the construction process. From ancient cultures through early-American barn-raisings, there is a tradition of whole towns gathering to put up a building. The combined advantages of low cost, speed, and conviviality make such work parties a tool for building community as well as structures. And the people who had a hand in making a place will always feel especially welcome there.

If you choose to undertake all or part of the work yourself, you will have an unequalled opportunity to put your heart into crafting the final experience. You will feel a personal connection to every piece you work on. You will be right there to watch the place take form and to see unanticipated opportunities as they arise. You will be strengthening and exercising your body as you make something useful and enduring—a rare experience today. You will be uniting head and hands in a common goal.

---

[1]Dorothea Theodoratus, "Preserving the Point Arena Roundhouse," *News From Native California,* September/October, 1987, p. 5.

You will also be exposing yourself to smashed thumbs, pulled muscles, back pain, and the dust and fumes of construction. The joys of building come with cautions. You could damage your health even before you move into your new healing environment.

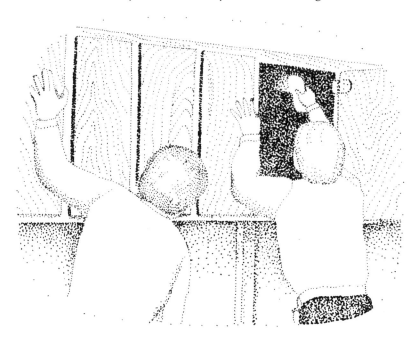

Know your limits, learn the proper use of tools, and don't try to prove how tough you are.

It's okay to take construction slowly. In the days of cathedrals, temples, or pyramids, important structures were rarely finished in one person's lifetime; they were usually experienced in the process of becoming. Today, construction occurs relatively quickly; we tend to see it as a necessary evil to be gotten through in the interests of being finished.[2] You needn't take several lifetimes, but taking your time allows the process to be organic. It lets you make discoveries along the way, incorporate changes, and respond to new insights. For example, you may not know what the views are like from the second floor until the floor is in place;

---

[2]The structure of taxes and loans often encourages rapid construction. If it is important to you to take your time, make sure your financial arrangements are geared to that.

why make final decisions on window placement before then? In many ways, being in and around a building as it goes up allows you to get to know it much better than you did when it was in your head or on paper. There's no better time for seeing and incorporating new ideas.[3]

BUILDING HEALTH

No matter how small or large the project, every aspect of it from the initial desire through planning, building, and moving in contributes to the healthfulness of the place. Intentions, choices made, emotions invested, and muscles applied all reside in the final product. Your investment in healing environments will pay off in increased energy and happiness, decreased medical bills, and less need for expensive escapes from unpleasant surroundings. Building for health needn't cost more than ordinary construction or decorating. But failing to alter an unhealthy environment might be expensive in the long run.

RESOURCES

The Place of Houses by Charles Moore, Gerald Allen, and Donlyn Lyndon; Holt, Rinehart and Winston, 1974.

How to Design and Build Your Own House by Lupe DiDonno and Phyllis Sperling; Alfred A. Knopf, 1985.

The Owner-Built Home by Ken Kern; Charles Scribner's Sons, 1975.

Before You Build (1981) and *Building Your Own House* (1984) by Robert Roskind; Ten Speed Press.

---

[3]Your local Building Department, which will have issued you a permit to build according to drawings you submitted, and your General Contractor, who may have given you a bid based on the same drawings, may or may not be happy to go along with such an approach. In some cases, changes may even require re-engineering. But if you plan for flexibility and communicate with your architect, engineer, and builder about it, you should be able to overcome potential obstacles.

Your Home, Your Health, and Well-Being by David Rousseau, Ten Speed Press, 1988.

The Motion-Minded Kitchen by Sam Clark; Houghton Mifflin Company, 1983.

A Pattern Language by Christopher Alexander et al; Oxford University Press, 1977.

The Moveable Nest by Tom Schneider; Ten Speed Press, 1984.

Fine Homebuilding magazine; The Taunton Press, 63 South Main Street, P.O. Box 355, Newtown, CT 06470.

Rodale's *Practical Homeowner,* P.O. Box 6020, Emmaus, PA 18098-0620.

Home magazine; P.O. Box 56318, Boulder, CO 80322-6318.

Ask your librarian or bookseller for guidance to many other excellent publications.

· CHAPTER · 17 ·

Conclusion and Beginning

*To be healthy ourselves we must heal the Earth
and create an environment in which the nurture of that
which sustains life is a constant goal.*
—MIKE SAMUELS & HAL BENNETT

In reading this book, you have begun a journey that will last the rest of your life. As with any inner search or effort to learn and grow via a relationship with something outside ourselves, there will always be new adventures and new subtleties to discover.

You are probably now in a different environment than you were in when you started reading this book, simply by virtue of your changed perceptions. As you continue to expand your awareness, enhance your environment, and improve your health, you will have increasing levels of clarity and energy to imagine a better life—and to make it happen.

The more you trust your perceptions, the more clearly you will see not only the places where you live and work, but every place you go. The more you conceive and carry out projects that improve your physical environment, the more you will feel capable of influencing other areas for the better. And the more you expand your awareness of the interconnectedness of all things, the more deeply you will know that indoor health is not an isolated issue—that indoor air and noise pollution are intimately linked to outdoor pollution, and that fragmentation and lack of self-determination are a source of ill health throughout our culture.

You will probably become more acutely aware of ways in which your neighborhood, city, bioregion, country, and planet need healing. Your successes with your immediate environment will convince you that you have the ability to set changes in motion. Your increased vitality—a part of the healthful actions you take—will assure you that there is something worth working for: a level of joy and involvement in life that most of us don't even know is possible.

It is healthy to be alarmed at the declining vitality of our planet and the potential for the end of all life via nuclear holocaust. But the best workers for peace and ecological sanity are those who have deeply touched their own wholeness, who have loved themselves well enough to love the world, and who give themselves a home base that nourishes their own physical, mental, and spiritual vitality. Taking care of yourself is not selfish; it is a gift to all of life.

Health requires balance between inner and outer, between activity and repose. It requires mental adaptability. And, most of all, it requires hope.

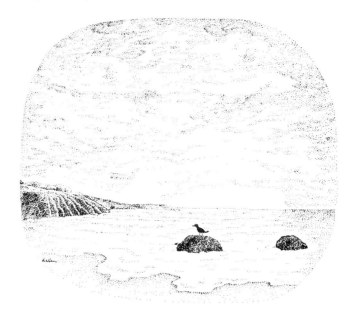

Progress is possible only when people believe in the possibilities of growth and change. Races or tribes die out not just when they are conquered and suppressed but when they accept their defeated condition, become despairing, and lose their excitement about the future . . .

There is no single formula for human survival, but the approach to survival has two main elements. The first is that we ought never to minimize or underestimate the nature of the problems that confront us. The second is that we ought never to minimize or underestimate our ability to deal with them. Human potentiality is the least understood and most squandered resource on earth. So long as human beings are capable of growth—intellectual, spiritual, and philosophical—they have a chance, a very good chance.

—Norman Cousins

· BIBLIOGRAPHY ·

Achterberg, Jeanne. *Imagery in Healing: Shamanism and Modern Medicine.* Boston: New Science Library/Shambhala, 1985.

Adair, Margo. *Working Inside Out: Tools for Change.* Berkeley: Wingbow Press, 1984.

Adelman, Dennis, "Radiant-Floor Heating." *Fine Homebuilding.* August/September, 1984, pp. 68-71.

Alexander, Christopher; Ishikawa, Sara; and Silverstein, Murray. *A Pattern Language.* New York: Oxford University Press, 1977.

American Public Health Association, Inc. *Principles for Healthful Rural Housing.* New York: American Public Health Association, Inc., 1957.

Andelman, Julian B., "Inhalation Exposure in the Home to Volatile Organic Contaminants of Drinking Water." *The Science of the Total Environment.* Amsterdam: Elsevier Science Publishers B.V., 1985.

Anderson, Richard feather, "Divining the Spirit of Place." *Yoga Journal.* September/October, 1986, pp. 27-31, 56-59.

Aranyi, Laszlow, and Goldman, Larry L. *Design of Long-Term Care Facilities.* New York: Van Nostrand Reinhold Company, 1980.

Ardalan, Nader, and Bakhtiar, Laleh. *The Sense of Unity: The Sufi Tradition in Persian Architecture.* Chicago: The University of Chicago Press, 1973.

Ardell, Donald B. *High Level Wellness.* Emmaus, Pennsylvania: Rodale Press, 1977.

Bender, Tom. *Environmental Design Primer.* Salem, Oregon: Published by the author, 1973.

_____."Putting Heart Into Our Homes." *Yoga Journal.* September/October, 1986, pp. 38-41, 50-51.

Bethards, Betty. *Techniques for Health and Wholeness.* Novato, California: Inner Light Foundation, 1979.

Birren, Faber. *Light, Color, and Environment*. New York: Van Nostrand Reinhold Company, 1982.

——————. "The Significance of Light: Reactions of Mind and Emotion." *AIA Journal*. October, 1972, pp. 37-40.

Blakeslee, Sandra, "Buildings That Make You Sick." *San Francisco Chronicle*. June 15, 1980, p. 3.

Bruce, Gene. "The Bedroom Goes Natural." *East West*, March, 1987, pp. 56-59.

California Department of Consumer Affairs. *Clean Your Room!* Sacramento: California Department of Consumer Affairs, 1982.

Canter, David, and Canter, Sandra. *Designing for Therapeutic Environments*. Chichester: John Wiley & Sons, 1979.

Carey, Deborah Allen. *Hospice Inpatient Environments*. New York: Van Nostrand Reinhold Company, 1986.

Carlisle, Norman, and Carlisle, Madelyn. *Where to Live for Your Health*. New York: Harcourt Brace Jovanovich, 1980.

Cavendish, Richard, ed. *Man, Myth, and Magic*. New York: Marshall Cavendish Corporation, 1970.

Chahroudi, Day. "Biosphere." *Mother Earth News*, December, 1972, center poster.

Clark, Linda. *The Ancient Art of Color Therapy*. New York: Pocket Books, 1975.

Cooper, Clare. "The House as Symbol of the Self." *Designing for Human Behavior*. Edited by Jon Lang. Stroudsburg, Pennsylvania: Dowden, Hutchinson, and Ross, Inc., 1974.

Cooper, Patricia, and Cook, Laurel. *Hot Springs and Spas of California*. San Francisco: 101 Productions, 1978.

Cousins, Norman. *Anatomy of an Illness*. New York: W.W. Norton & Company, 1979.

Crane, Catherine C. *Personal Places*. New York: Whitney Library of Design, 1982.

Crook, William G., M.D. *The Yeast Connection.* Jackson, Tennessee, Professional Books, 1984.

Dadd, Debra Lynn. "The All-Natural House, An Interview With Paul Bierman-Lytle." *Everything Natural,* September/October, 1986, pp. 10-13.

——————. "Basic Toxicology." *Everything Natural,* January/February, 1987, pp. 15-17.

——————. "The Beauty of Nature in Your Home." *Everything Natural,* July/August, 1987, pp. 15-18.

——————. "Less-Toxic Building Materials, An Interview With Mary Oetzel." *Everything Natural,* September/October, pp. 16-17.

——————. "Book Review: *Light, Radiation, and You.*" *Everything Natural,* September/October, 1985, p. 9.

——————. *Nontoxic and Natural.* Los Angeles: Jeremy P. Tarcher, Inc., 1984.

——————. *The Nontoxic Home.* Los Angeles: Jeremy P. Tarcher, Inc., 1986.

——————. "Sound Health: An Interview With Steven Halpern on Sound and Wellness." *Everything Natural,* July/August, 1986, pp. 1-8.

Davis, Steven Andrew, M.D. *How to Stay Healthy in an Unhealthy World.* New York: William Morrow and Company, Inc., 1983.

Deliman, Tracy, and Smolowe, John S., M.D. *Holistic Medicine: Harmony of Body, Mind, Spirit.* Reston, Virginia: Reston Publishing Company, Inc., A Prentice-Hall Company, 1982.

Diamond, Harvey, and Diamond, Marilyn. *Fit For Life.* New York: Warner Books, 1985.

Dubos, Rene. "The Biological Basis of Urban Design." *Ekistics,* April, 1973, pp. 199-204.

——————. *Man Adapting.* New Haven: Yale University Press, 1965.

——————. *The Wooing of Earth.* New York: Charles Scribner's Sons, 1980.

Duhl, Leonard J., M.D. and Den Boer, James. *Making Whole: Health for a New Epoch.* Manuscript, University California, Berkeley, 1980.

—————————. *Health Planning and Social Change.* New York: Human Sciences Press, Inc., 1986.

"Electricity, Conduction of." *Encyclopaedia Britannica.* 1965. Vol. 8, p. 202.

Ember, Lois. "EPA Compiling Data on Extent of Indoor Radon Hazard." *Chemical & Engineering News,* August 17, 1987, pp. 22-24.

"EPA Finds Radon a Widespread Health Threat." *Chemical & Engineering News,* August 10, 1987, p. 18.

Evans, Benjamin H., A.I.A. *Daylight in Architecture.* New York: Architectural Record Books, McGraw Hill Book Company, 1981.

Fanger. P. O. and Valbjorn, O., eds. *Indoor Climate.* Copenhagen: Danish Building Research Institute, 1979.

Farr, Lee E., "Medical Consequences of Environmental Home Noises." *People and Buildings.* Edited by Robert Gutman. New York: Basic Books, Inc., 1972.

Fast, Julius. *Weather Language.* New York: Wyden Books, distrubuted by Simon & Schuster, 1979.

Fawcett, Howard H. "Air Pollution Indoors." *Chemical and Engineering News,* January 19, 1987, pp. 48-49.

Fitch, James Marston. *American Building: The Environmental Forces That Shape it.* New York: Schocken Books, 1972.

Flynn, John E., and Segil, Arthur W. *Architectural Interior Systems.* New York: Van Nostrand Reinhold Company, 1970.

Fossel, Peter. "Sick-Home Blues." *Harrowsmith,* September/October, 1987, pp. 46-55, 135.

Foster, Lee. "Creating Your Own Backyard Wildlife Sanctuary." *Friendly Exchange.* Spring, 1981, pp. 20-23.

Garfield, Patricia, Ph.D. *Creative Dreaming.* New York: Ballantine Books, 1974.

Gehrig, Franciska. *House Your Soul.* San Francisco: Published by the author, 465 Brussels, 94134.

Goromosov, M.S. *The Physiological Basis of Health Standards for Dwellings*. Geneva: World Health Organization, 1968.

Hall, Edward T., "Let's Heat People Instead of Houses." *Human Nature*. January, 1979, pp. 45-47.

Halpern, Steven. *Sound Health*. San Francisco: Harper & Row, 1985.

Harker, Charles. "Psychosynergetic Space." 1975. (mimeographed).

Hastings, Arthur C., Ph.D.; Fadiman, James, Ph.D.; and Gordon, James S., M.D., eds. *Health for the Whole Person*. Boulder, Colorado: Westview Press, 1980.

Heschong, Lisa. *Thermal Delight in Architecture*. Cambridge, Massachusetts: The M.I.T. Press, 1979.

Hinkle, Lawrence E., Jr., M.D., and Loring, William C., Ph.D., eds. *The Effect of the Man-Made Environment on Health and Behavior*. United States Department of Health, Education, and Welfare, Publication No. (CDC) 77-8318.

Hodgkinson, Neville. *Will to be Well*. York Beach, Maine: Samuel Weiser, Inc., 1984.

Holborn, Mark. *The Ocean in the Sand: Japan From Landscape to Garden*. Boulder, Colorado: Shambhala, 1978.

Ismael, Cristina. *The Healing Environment*. Millbrae, California: Celestial Arts, 1976.

Jaffe, Dennis T., Ph.D. *Healing From Within*. New York: A Fireside Book, Published by Simon & Schuster, Inc., 1986.

Jayne, Walter Addison, M.D. *The Healing Gods of Ancient Civilizations*. New York: University Books, 1962 (first published in 1925).

Jemmott, John B., III, and Locke, Steven, M.D. "Psychosocial Factors, Immunological Mediation, and Human Susceptibility to Infectious Diseases: How Much Do We Know?" *Psychological Bulletin*, Vol. 95, No. 1. (1984), 78-108.

Jones, Alex. *Seven Mansions of Color*. Marina del Rey, California: DeVorss & Company, 1982.

Kane, Leslie, "The Power of Color." *Health*. July, 1982, pp. 36-39.

Kern, Ken. *The Owner-Built Home.* New York: Charles Scribner's Sons, 1975.

Kodama, Yuichiro. "A House for all Seasons." Paper presented at the Environmental Evolution and Technologies Conference, University of Texas at Austin, August, 1975.

Kohler, Mariane, and Chapelle, Jean. *101 Recipes for Sound Sleep.* New York: Walker and Company, 1965.

Kron, Joan. *Home-Psych.* New York: Clarkson N. Potter, Inc., Publishers, 1983.

Krueger, Albert P. and Sigel, Sheelah. "Ions in the Air," *Human Nature,* July, 1978, pp. 46-52.

Kushi, Michio. *How To See Your Health: Book of Oriental Diagnosis.* New York: Japan Publications, Inc., 1980.

La Favore, Michael. "The Radon Report." *Rodale's New Shelter,* January, 1986, pp. 29-35.

Lamb, Curt. *Homestyles.* New York: St. Martin's Press, 1979.

Lindheim, Roslyn, and Chater, Shirley S. *Symposium on Environments for Humanized Health Care.* Berkeley: University of California, 1979.

Locke, Steven E., M.D. "Stress, Adaptation, and Immunity: Studies in Humans." *General Hospital Psychiatry,* 4 (1982), pp. 49-58.

Lohmeier, Lynne, Ph.D., "Indoor Pollution Alert." *East West.* March, 1987, pp. 42-47.

—————————. "Let the Sun Shine In." *East West.* July, 1986, pp. 36-43.

Lourie, Reginald S. "Consideration for the Young in a City for Human Development." *Ekistics,* April, 1973, pp. 220-223.

Luttrell, Michael. "Warm Floors." *Fine Homebuilding.* June/July, 1985, pp. 68-77.

McDonald, Elvin. *Plants as Therapy.* New York: Praeger Publishers, 1976.

Mandell, Marshall, M.D. *Dr. Mandell's 5-Day Allergy Relief System.* New York: Pocket Books, 1979.

March, Andrew L. "The Winds, the Waters and the Living *Qi.*" *Parabola,* Vol. III, Issue 1, 1978, pp. 28-34.

Neihardt, John G. *Black Elk Speaks*. New York: Washington Square Books, 1959.

Olgyay, Victor. *Design With Climate*. Princeton, New Jersey: Princeton University Press, 1963.

Ott, John N. *Health and Light*. New York: Pocket Books, 1976.

Palmer, Bruce. *Body Weather*. New York: Jove/HBJ Books, 1976.

Pfeiffer, Guy O., and Nikel, Casimir M., eds. *The Household Environment and Chronic Illness*. Springfield, Illinois: Charles C. Thomas, Publisher, 1980.

Potts, Eve, and Morra, Marion. *Understanding Your Immune System*. New York: Avon Books, 1986.

Randegger, Suzanne. "Focus on Light." *Environ*. Winter 1985-86, pp. 14-16, 18-20.

──────────, and Randegger, Ed. "A Real Rocky Mountain High?" *Environ*. Fall-Winter, 1986-87, p. 23.

──────────. "Formaldehyde and Health." *Environ*. Fall-Winter 1986-87, pp. 6-12.

──────────. "HRVs Help Reduce Home Pollution." *Environ*. Fall-Winter, 1986-87, p. 19.

──────────. "Radon: A Natural Killer." *Environ*. Fall-Winter, pp. 14-17.

──────────. "Q & A Dept." *Environ*. Summer, 1985, p. 23.

Robinette, Gary O. *Plants/People/and Environmental Quality*. Washington, D.C.: U.S. Department of the Interior, National Park Service, 1972.

Rossbach, Sarah. *Feng Shui: The Chinese Art of Placement*. New York: E.P. Dutton, Inc., 1983.

Rousseau, David; Rea, W.J., M.D.; and Enwright, Jean. *Your Home, Your Health, and Well-Being*. Berkeley: Ten Speed Press, 1988.

Ryan, Regina Sara, and Travis, John W., M.D. *The Wellness Workbook*. Berkeley: Ten Speed Press, 1981.

Saifer, Mark, Ph.D. "Negative Ions: 'Vitamins of the Air' or 'Hot Air'?" *The Human Ecologist,* December, 1979, p. 6.

Samuels, Mike, M.D., and Bennett, Hal. *The Well Body Book*. New York: Random House/Bookworks, 1973.

Selye, Hans, M.D. *The Stress of Life*. New York: McGraw Hill Book Co., 1976.

Small, Bruce. "Creating Your Own Safe Environment." *Environ*. Fall, 1985, pp. 4-6.

Spence, Michael D. "Water." *Environ*, No. 6.

Theodoratus, Dorothea. "Preserving the Point Arena Roundhouse." *News From Native California*, September/October, 1987, pp. 4-5.

Todd, Nancy Jack, and Todd, John. *Bioshelters, Ocean Arks, City Farming: Ecology as the Basis of Design*. San Francisco: Sierra Club Books, 1984.

Turiel, Isaac. *Indoor Air Quality and Human Health*. Stanford, California: Stanford University Press, 1985.

Ullman, Montague, M.D., and Zimmerman, Nan. *Working With Dreams*. New York: Delacorte Press/Eleanor Friede, 1979.

"Visiting Japan's Housing 'Parks'." *Sunset*. December, 1986.

Watts, May Theilgaard. *Reading the Landscape*. New York: The MacMillan Company, 1957.

Wilkens, Emily. *Secrets From the Super Spas*. New York: Grosset & Dunlap, 1976.

Wood, Betty. *The Healing Power of Color*. New York: Destiny Books, 1984.

Wurtman, Richard J. "Biological Considerations in Lighting Environments." *Progressive Architecture*, September, 1973, pp. 79-81.

Zamm, Alfred V., M.D., with Gannon, Robert. *Why Your House May Endanger Your Health*. New York: A Touchstone Book, Published by Simon and Schuster, 1980.

· INDEX ·

A

Absorption of sound, 94
Adair, Margo, 17
Adobe, as building material, 121
Aerosol sprays, as pollution source,
114-115
"Aesculapia," 185-187
Air
See also Ventilation
for healing centers, 189
for relaxation space, 155
for sleep environment, 143-145,
146
in workplace, 154, 155
Air conditioning
disadvantages of, 77
health and, 13, 72
historical perspective, 70
noise and, 88, 93
recommendations for, 77-78
Air exchange
with radiant heating, 82
ventilation and, 118
Air filtration, 120
for formaldehyde protection, 104
for house dust protection, 110
for radon protection, 108
Air fresheners, as pollution source,
114
Air ions, 112-114
Alexander, Christopher, 136, 150,
151, 184
Allergies, house dust, 109-110
plants, 135. *See also*
Environmental sensitivity
Ambient noise, 85-89
avoiding, 90-91

Ambient vs. radiant heating, 79-80,
81-82
Analogous colors, 61
Anderson, Richard feather, 173
Animal hair, in house dust, 109-110
Appliances
isolating and venting, 117, 119
as noise source, 87, 88, 93
as pollution source, 105-106
Ardalan, Nader, 61
Asbestos, 109, 126
Awareness, 23-29
in children, 32-33
passive heating or cooling and, 73-
75
Awareness exercises
childhood impressions, 30-32
color, 62-63
how to use, 5-6
imaginary healing place, 28-29
lighting, 54-55
noticing the environment, 23
outdoor environment, 137
place energy, 172-173
present and imaged environments,
16
self and home, 37
sonic environment, 89-90
symbolic meanings, 41-42
thermal environment, 71, 83
using, 192

B

Backyard Wildlife Habitat Program,
135
Bacteria, in house dust, 109-110

Carol Venolia is an architect with a longstanding interest in the relationship between life and buildings. Through her architectural practice on the Mendocino/Sonoma coast, she designs buildings, consults, writes, lectures, and gives workshops nationally. She welcomes tales of your experiences with healing environments. She also publishes a newsletter, *Building with Nature*. For subscription information, write to P.O. Box 369, Gualala, CA 95445.